B. L. Grundy and R. M. Villani (eds.)

Evoked Potentials

*Intraoperative
and ICU Monitoring*

Springer-Verlag Wien New York

Betty L. Grundy

Professor of Anesthesiology, University of Florida, College of Medicine, and
Chief Anesthesiology Service, Veterans Administration Medical Center,
Gainesville, Fla., U.S.A.

Roberto M. Villani

Professor and Chairman, Institute of Neurosurgery, University of Milano, Milano,
Italy

© 1988 by Springer-Verlag/Wien

Printed in Austria

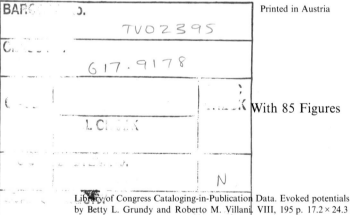

With 85 Figures

Library of Congress Cataloging-in-Publication Data. Evoked potentials: intraoperative and ICU monitoring/edited
by Betty L. Grundy and Roberto M. Villani. VIII, 195 p. 17.2 × 24.3 cm. ISBN 0-387-82059-0 (U.S.) 1. Evoked
potentials (Electrophysiology). 2. Surgery—Physiological aspects. 3. Patient monitoring. 4. Intensive care units.
I. Grundy, Betty L. II. Villani, R. RD52.E85E96 1988. 617'.9178-dc19. 88-20173

ISBN 3-211-82059-0 Springer-Verlag Wien New York
ISBN 0-387-82059-0 Springer-Verlag New York Wien

Foreword

In June 1986, the Institute of Neurosurgery, University of Milano, with the generous help of Amplifon SpA, organized an international symposium on the use of evoked potentials for monitoring nervous functions during surgical procedures and in treating patients admitted to intensive care units.

We are personally convinced that this monitoring technique has definite and objective validity; we wanted to compare our experience with that of other groups working in the field to confirm our data and, if possible, to extend applications to other areas. The possibility of knowing during a surgical operation whether the procedures we perform are in themselves harmless or dangerous is an irreplaceable help in the progress of neuro-surgical technique. Evoked potential monitoring appears to be specific and reliable, unlike other methods of nervous system monitoring that were available in the past. In fact, the evaluation of neurological signs is nec-essarily very scanty during anesthesia and intraoperative electroencepha-lography is highly aspecific. It was mandatory to compare different ex-periences from all over the world, in order to assess the reliability of intraoperative evoked potential monitoring, its possible applications and its limitations.

As concerns head-injured patients in the intensive care unit, needed is a diagnostic tool more precise than clinical evaluation (which is always subjective) and therefore able to forecast more correctly the final outcome of patients; this requirement has been partially fulfilled by the use of evoked potential monitoring in clinical routine.

This book collects most of the contributions presented in the Symposium on Evoked Potential Monitoring, that, according to participants, was ex-tremely stimulating and successful. The chapters treat the same topics discussed in the meeting.

The book is addressed to all clinicians and researchers dealing with the evaluation of nervous function in comatose patients and in patients sub-jected to surgery of either the central nervous system or the main arteries supplying it.

A special acknowledgement is due to Dr. Grundy for many reasons. First she prompted research in the field of evoked potential monitoring with her pioneering papers; second, she joined us in the meeting, which allowed us to match our work with her wide experience; and last, but not

least, she did an incredible and exhausting work in reviewing all the manu-
scripts included in this book.

Finally, I would like to thank Dr. Ducati for his invaluable cooperation:
he started the technique of evoked potentials in our institute and organized
the symposium, with the help of his young colleagues Dr. E. Fava, Dr. M.
Cenzato and Dr. A. Landi. Without them neither the symposium nor this
book would have ever seen the light.

Dr. Roberto Villani
Professor and Chairman
Institute of Neurosurgery
University of Milano
President of the Symposium

Contents

EEG and Evoked Potentials: Rationale for ICU Recording and Monitoring

R. Q. Cracco

State University of New York Health Science Center at Brooklyn, Department
of Neurology, Brooklyn, New York (U.S.A.)

Recording or monitoring the EEG or evoked potentials (EPs) in the ICU provides useful information in acutely neurologically ill patients whenever a relationship exists between the electrical activity and the (1) functional integrity of CNS structures; (2) clinical status; (3) diagnosis or (4) prognosis. In brain death such a correlation is clearly present. In certain countries, including Italy, an EEG is required by law before a diagnosis of brain death can be made and donor organs removed. In other countries, including the United Kingdom and the United States, the diagnosis of brain death can be made on clinical grounds alone, although an EEG is often obtained to confirm this diagnosis. A clinical diagnosis of brain death requires demonstrating the absence of brain and brainstem function when depressant drug intoxication and hypothermia can be excluded. Hypothermia poses no problem since the patient can be warmed and the examination repeated. Excluding the presence of depressant drugs is more difficult. Electrocerebral inactivity or electrocerebral silence which is consistent with a clinical diagnosis of brain death is defined as no EEG activity over $2\,\mu V$ when recording from scalp electrode pairs 10 or more cm apart with interelectrode impedances under 10,000 ohms but over 100 ohms. The value of $2\,\mu V$ was selected because many EEG machines have noise levels of up to $2\,\mu V$. The EEG is often recorded with difficulty in the electrically hostile environment of the ICU. It is imperative that technicians are well trained, taught to apply electrodes with care, and identify, and, when possible, eliminate artifact. Ten guidelines recommended by the American EEG Society for EEG recordings in cases of suspected cerebral death are:

(1) a minimum of 8 scalp electrodes should be utilized; (2) interelectrode impedances should be under 10,000 ohms but over 100 ohms; (3) the integrity of the entire recording system should be tested such as by touching each electrode of the montage; (4) interelectrode distances should be at

least 10 cm; (5) sensitivity must be increased to at least $2 \mu V/mm$ for at least 30 minutes of the recording with inclusion of appropriate calibrations; (6) filter settings should be appropriate; (7) additional monitoring techniques should be employed when necessary (*e.g.*, EKG, respiration, movements, etc); (8) there should be no EEG reactivity to intense somatosensory, auditory or visual stimuli; (9) recordings should be made only by a qualified technologist; (10) a repeat EEG should be performed if there is doubt about electrocerebral silence.

Electrocerebral silence can be recorded in patients who are not brain dead. Such patients are usually hypothermic, drug intoxicated or in a persistent vegetative state with irreversible destruction of cerebral cortex but with preserved brainstem function. Additionally, the EEG is not consistently reliable in confirming the diagnosis of brain death in young children under 6 years of age. In young patients and patients of all ages suspected of depressant drug intoxication, brainstem auditory evoked potentials (BAEPs) and short latency somatosensory evoked potentials (SSEPs) provide useful information. Only BAEP Wave I (and rarely II) and SSEP components N 9, N 11, N 13 and P 13–14 are present in brain dead patients. Conversely, BAEP and SSEP components are all present and normal or only slightly increased in interpeak latency in patients with depressant drug intoxication even when EEG shows electrocerebral silence.

Evoked potentials and the EEG are often of value in comatose or unresponsive patients. An EEG diagnosis of alpha coma can be made on the basis of the presence of nonreactive EEG activity of alpha frequency which is generalized though usually maximal at anterior scalp recording locations. The prognosis is usually poor in such patients. This EEG pattern must be distinguished from the normal posteriorly distributed reactive alpha activity which is seen in some patients who are "locked in" and from drug induced fast activity that can be slowed to alpha frequency. Drug induced alpha frequency activity is often maximal at anterior scalp recording locations and may be superimposed on slower delta frequency activity. As drug induced coma increases in severity, suppression burst activity is recorded which may be followed by potentially reversible electrocerebral silence.

It is important to identify electrographic seizure discharges in EEGs performed on unresponsive patients. Epileptic status can be subclinical and treatment of the epilepsy can be life saving. Burst suppression activity is often recorded in comatose patients. This pattern usually implies a poor prognosis except when it is caused by acute drug intoxication.

Comatose patients whose EEG demonstrates varying sleep-like patterns usually have a better prognosis than those with unchanging sleep-like patterns (see Bricolo – this volume). The occurrence of "triphasic" waves in the EEG of a stuporous patient should suggest the possibility of a metabolic disturbance such as uremia or hepatic encephalopathy. Focal abnormalities such as delta focus or periodic lateralized epileptiform discharges indicate a focal lesion. The latter pattern is usually associated with acute or subacute lesions of vascular or infectious origin, and an underlying metabolic disorder is frequently present. Herpes infection is often found in young patients whose EEG is characterized by this discharge.

Pattern shift visual evoked potentials (PSVEPs) are infrequently useful in the neurological ICU. This is because PSVEPs require the patient's cooperation which is not possible in many acutely ill neurological patients. BAEPs and SSEPs do not require the patient's cooperation. SSEPs and BAEPs are very resistant to toxic or metabolic conditions. In evaluating these EPs in patients with CNS disease it is important that peripheral structures such as auditory and peripheral nerves are intact. This can be verified by identifying BAEP I which is generated in the auditory nerve and by recording over median nerve fibers at Erb's point and measuring BAEP and SSEP interpeak latencies. Barbiturate levels twice those required to give electrocerebral silence result in BAEPs and SSEPs which have normal or only slightly increased interpeak latencies. These EPs are therefore useful in monitoring head trauma patients undergoing high dose barbiturate therapy for increased intracranial pressure. In these comatose patients the clinical evaluation provides limited information and the EEG may reveal electrocerebral silence. Conversely, when there is structural pathology, then both BAEPs and SSEPs are likely to be abnormal. In patients with pontine midbrain haemorrhage, BAEP components I, II and III are preserved, while IV and V are usually absent. Similarly, SSEP component N 20 is usually absent in these patients whereas earlier components are present. Rostral pontine or mesencephalic lesions may give increased BAEP I–V and SSEP N 13 or $P_{13—14}$-N 20 interpeak latencies. BAEPs are usually not useful in patients with supratentorial lesions since shifts in brain structure rather than increased intracranial pressure per se seem to cause abnormal BAEPs. Hence the brainstem structures which generate these components are affected only very late with supratentorial lesions at a time when the prognosis is poor. Conversely, SSEPs are useful in patients with supratentorial lesions since the N 20 and P 23 components are generated in somesthetic cortex and may be absent or increased in peak latency.

The SSEP has been found to be of great utility in judging prognosis in comatose patients. Like BAEPs these are altered by structural pathology and are relatively unaffected by metabolic or toxic conductions. When N 20 is absent bilaterally (with independent stimulation of both the left and the right median nerves) the patients almost invariably die or enter into a persistent vegetative state when the underlying pathology is due to hypoxia or ischemia. If N 20 is absent unilaterally and hemiparesis is present at the time of the recording, then the hemiparesis is likely to persist. Finally, if N 20 is present bilaterally, the prognosis is good and the patients also usually look good clinically. Recently, Symons found that increased SSEP central conduction time (N 20-N 13 interpeak latency difference) is correlated with decreased cerebral blood flow.

Greenberg has studied multimodality EPs (cortical VEPs and cortical and subcortical auditory and somatosensory EPs) in patients with acute closed head injury. Patients in whom only subcortical EPs were recorded invariably died or entered a persistent vegetative state. The majority of patients with recordable EPs of cortical origin survived but often with varying degrees of neurological impairment.

The integrity of spinal cord afferent pathways can be studied by recording SSEPs to stimulation of nerves in the lower extremities from electrodes placed on the scalp. Abnormalities of these potentials have been observed in patients with spinal cord pathology of many types, including spinal cord trauma. It is well established that failure to record any scalp potential correlates with physiological transection of the spinal cord afferent pathways which contribute to the scalp potential. Most of these patients have clinically evident complete spinal cord lesions and poor prognosis. Conversely, the recording of a scalp response rules out cord transection and the prognosis in many of these patients is good. Although the diagnosis of a complete cord lesion can usually be reliably made on clinical grounds alone, scalp recorded SSEPs provide valuable information in patients where the clinical exam is unreliable, such as in confused, demented or very young patients. Patients with cord trauma may have impaired mental status because of associated head injuries. The recording of scalp SSEPs is presently of limited value in monitoring patients with acute spinal cord injury. One reason for this is that specific criteria for defining significant changes in SSEP, aside from complete absence of a scalp potential, have not been established.

The recording of spinal SSEPs from surface electrodes placed over the spine has also provided useful information about the conduction characteristics of spinal afferent pathways in children, adults and patients with certain diseases of the spinal cord. The major problem with this noninvasive method is technical. Responses recorded over rostral cord segments in adults are very small and failure to record such potentials cannot be regarded as abnormal since they cannot be obtained in some normal subjects. The method of obtaining spine-scalp propagation velocities by recording SSEPs over both spine and scalp can be expected to provide useful and quantitative information in patients with spinal cord and other diseases affecting the spinal cord. The technical problem of difficulty in recording potentials from rostral spine leads is eliminated by recording potentials from more caudal spinal locations where the potentials can be reliably obtained and from the scalp. The narrow standard deviations obtained with this method suggest it is sensitive and will prove valuable in assessing patients with incomplete spinal cord lesions.

Intensive longterm ICU evoked potential monitoring is difficult and much must be done to improve this methodology. Identification of an EP change which occurs during monitoring and which is associated with irreversible neurologic impairment is of little value to the patient. Detection of reversible change which can affect the management of the patient and result in avoiding complications is the objective of monitoring. The problem is that significant reversible EP changes are difficult to identify and precisely define. If modifying a treatment because of an EP change results in a good outcome, one cannot conclude that the treatment necessarily affected the outcome, since it is a fact that EP changes which occur when no change in treatment is carried out may also result in a good outcome. Similarly, when treatment is modified because of an EP change a bad outcome may result. It is important that significant EP changes which indicate potentially reversible clinical deterioration are identified. Such EP changes should provide a low incidence of false positives and false negatives. A low incidence of false positives will avoid unnecessary and potentially harmful medical intervention. Similarly a low incidence of false negatives is also important; otherwise indicated medical intervention which may avoid complications will not be undertaken. The most common cause of false negatives in EP monitoring is failure to monitor the appropriate neural structures such as monitoring sensory evoked potentials in patients who develop abnormalities in motor function.

Effective ICU EP monitoring must sometimes be carried out 24 hours a day for a period of many days. Trained technicians and physicians with a knowledge of electrophysiology must always be available. An automated system capable of identifying significant EP changes, as defined above, and rapidly reporting such changes to medical personnel has not yet been devised. Devising such a system should be a major goal in EP research.

In 1980 Merton and Morton devised a noninvasive method whereby single electrical stimuli were delivered to the scalp transcranially and motor action potentials were recorded from muscles of the upper and lower extremities. Initially the levels of stimulation used were very high and resulted in considerable patient discomfort. Subsequently, Hassan *et al.* devised a method which permitted more tolerable levels of stimulation. Recently Barker and his colleagues described a method which uses magnetic stimulation to deliver electrical pulses to the cortex, and this technique produces little in the way of patient discomfort.

Transcranial evoked motor action potentials have been recorded in patients by several groups of investigators including Marsden *et al.*, Murray and Mills and Rossini *et al.* Patients with focal CNS lesions of varied etiology have been investigated and it seems that this method provides useful and reliable information concerning transmission in central descending motor pathways. This method is likely to be of great clinical value in evaluating many patients including those acutely ill in the ICU. Levy has used this method to monitor the integrity of descending motor pathways during brain and spinal cord surgery. Much work is currently being directed toward defining the precise pathways which mediate this response and demonstrating that the method is safe. To date, no significant untoward effects have been observed using this technique.

Recently Lueders *et al.* introduced a technique which consists of implanting chronically a large number of subdural electrodes over the epileptic focus of patients with epilepsy. These investigators attempted to precisely measure the extent of the epileptogenic focus and the functional capacity of the cortex at and immediately surrounding the focus. The objective was to permit excision of the focus in its entirety without resection of normal tissue essential for full functional capacity. A total of 64 subdural electrodes were placed in epileptic patients in the operating room. Patients were then returned to their rooms where recordings and certain tests were performed over the course of several days. Anticonvulsant medication was then withdrawn and additional recordings were performed. Using this technique, it is possible to map the sensorimotor area of the brain which is difficult to identify with certainty during surgery. One method which can be used to accomplish this is to record mu EEG activity which is largely localized to the hand area of the motor strip. SSEPs can also be recorded after stimulating the ring or index finger. These components are recorded as a horizontal dipole in the anterior-posterior direction. The subdural electrodes over the motor and sensory regions then record opposite ends of the dipole. However, this SSEP data must be interpreted with caution since the phase reversal sometimes occurs anterior to the Rolandic fissure. Delivering electrical stimuli to the cortex via the subdural electrodes and mapping motor and sensory regions provides the most useful and reliable information which can be obtained using this method. The exact motor and sensory regions involved in various functions vary considerably among subjects. Nevertheless, the extent of the motor and sensory strips can be precisely defined using this method so that the amount of cortical tissue that can be removed safely is identified. Lueders and his colleagues have mapped Wernicke's and Broca's speech areas and have identified a new speech area in the basal temporal region. Stimulation of the basal temporal speech area results in speech arrest without a disturbance of consciousness.

This review of some of the applications of EEG and EP recordings in patients in the ICU and in monitoring outside of the operating room demonstrates the increasing importance of these neurophysiologic techniques. In the ensuing decades such methods will be available at all major neurological centers.

References

1. Cracco RQ, Bodis-Wollner I (1986) Evoked potentials. Alan R Liss Inc, New York
2. Chiappa K (1983) Evoked potentials in clinical medicine. Raven Press, New York
3. Bodis-Wollner I (1982) Evoked potentials. Ann New York Acad Sci, pp 388
4. Hassan NF, Rossini PM, Cracco RQ, Cracco JB (1985) Unexposed motor cortex activation by low voltage stimuli. In: Morocutti C, Rizzo PA (eds) Evoked potentials: Neurophysiological and clinical aspects. Elsevier, Amsterdam, pp 107–113
5. Klass DW, Daly D (1979) Current practice of clinical electroencephalography. Raven Press, New York
6. Neurosurgery (Supplement on Motor Evoked Potentials). Jan 1987, Vol 20: 1
7. Journal of Clinical Neurophysiol (Supplement on Guidelines). Jan 1987
8. Lueders H et al (1986) Subdural electrodes. In: Engel J (ed) Surgical management of the epilepsies. Raven Press, New York
9. Young RR, Cracco RQ (1985) Clinical neurophysiology of conduction in central motor pathways. Ann Neurol 18: 606–610

Intraoperative Monitoring of Evoked Potentials

BETTY L. GRUNDY

Anesthesiology Service, Veterans Administration Medical Center, Gainesville, Florida (U.S.A.)

Evoked potentials (EPs), the electrophysiologic responses of the nervous system to stimulation, permit monitoring of the functional integrity of neurologic pathways when clinical monitoring is hampered by general anesthesia or coma. Intraoperative EP monitoring is now commonplace in many medical centers throughout the world. To use these techniques to best advantage, one must appreciate several important principles. This paper reviews key concepts in monitoring and describes key criteria for assessing EPs as monitors in the operating room. In conclusion, guidelines for avoiding "false positives" and "false negatives" are outlined.

Important Concepts in Monitoring

The Purpose of Intraoperative Monitoring

Many neurosurgeons have made important contributions to anesthesiology. For example, Harvey Cushing developed the anesthesia record while he was still a medical student. His initial experience with anesthesia was unfortunate. As the most junior member of the surgical team, he was asked to anesthetize a patient with a bowel obstruction. This was to be done with open drop ether in the hallway outside the operating theater. The patient vomited, aspirated, and died. Cushing was devastated. He went to his professor's home that evening, prepared to resign from medical school. The professor reassured him that this was actually quite common and that he should not be so concerned. Cushing then went on to study ways of improving the administration of anesthesia. Toward this end, he devised a chart showing the administration of anesthetic agents, pulse rate, and respiratory rate. He seems to have made a contribution to peer review in anesthesiology as well, since the chart was used to settle wagers with another student as to who had provided better anesthesia. Upon graduation from

medical school, he undertook a tour of Europe. In Italy, he saw Riva-
Rocci measure the blood pressure noninvasively by using a cuff. Thinking
that arterial blood pressure measurement would make a nice addition to
his anesthesia chart, Cushing returned to Boston and studied this measurement in a clinical series of patients. When he reported his data, the
more senior members of the medical school faculty determined that one
should not monitor the blood pressure during anesthesia, because it was
clearly too variable to be of any significance[1,2]. Three quarters of a century
later, no prospective randomized clinical trial has been performed to un-
equivocally show that monitoring of the arterial blood pressure makes a
global difference in outcomes of anesthesia care. It is not likely that such
a study will ever be conducted, but blood pressure monitoring is now widely,
if not universally, performed during anesthesia.

In the operating room, we do not look for measurements of physiologic
function that will guarantee bad outcomes. Instead, we do our best to
continually optimize function intraoperatively in the hopes of preventing
lasting damage during a period of recognized risk. Just as we cannot tell
what level of hypotension will guarantee a myocardial infarction or renal
failure in a given patient, we cannot always tell what abnormality in EPs
will guarantee a neurologic injury. We do know that if the blood pressure
or electrocardiographic signal is lost, as in cardiac arrest, the patient is
unlikely to do well unless the signal is restored. We also know that the
duration of cardiac arrest has an impact on prognosis, but an exact time-
table relating outcome to duration of arrest for the individual patient cannot
be described. Previously healthy patients have been reviewed after hours
of cardiac arrest when submerged in very cold water, while in other circumstances a patient may never regain consciousness after even a brief
cardiac arrest. Similarly, when EPs are lost intraoperatively, we know that
the prognosis for postoperative function in the monitored pathway is much
better if the EP signal can be restored well toward normal intraoperatively.
Thus, EP monitoring in the operating room or critical care unit differs
from the recordings performed in the clinical diagnostic laboratory. Intraoperatively, our mission is to continually optimize function to the greatest extent possible. The purposes of diagnosis and prognosis are of primary
concern in the diagnostic laboratory but are relatively less important than
optimization of function during clinical monitoring in the operating room
or critical care unit.

The Importance of Continuous Monitoring

Although the value of continuous monitoring during anesthesia has been
appreciated for many years, going back to early proponents of the constant
finger on the pulse still advocated by many, this principle is often neglected

by those who monitor EEG or EPs in the operating room. The expense and bother of keeping expensive equipment and highly trained personnel in the operating room probably explain much of this. For example, some clinicians monitor patients who have spine fusion for scoliosis only during distraction of the spine with Harrington rods or only during passage of sublaminar wires. Yet we know that spinal cord dysfunction can first appear at other points during the operation, particularly in the presence of hypotension, and that the onset of paraplegia may be as late as 48 hours after surgery[3].

In monitoring patients during carotid endarterectomy, some workers monitor EEG or EPs only during the period of carotid occlusion. Only a small proportion of the brain injuries related to carotid endarterectomy occur during the period of vessel occlusion, however. Most perioperative injuries are thought to be due to artery-to-artery embolism. In a series of 359 carotid endarterectomies performed with regional anesthesia, only 4% failed to tolerate carotid occlusion without a shunt[4]. Nevertheless, neurologic deficits lasting more than 24 hours were seen in 1.7% and deficits resolving within 24 hours were seen in an additional 4.3%. Only one (0.3%) was related to cerebral ischemia during carotid occlusion. Of the six deficits lasting more than 24 hours and the 15 lasting less than 24 hours, three developed during carotid dissection, two during release of carotid occlusion, and 15 during the first five postoperative days.

Changes in BAEPs[5, 6] or in SEPs[7] have been documented with changes in position during anesthesia, and these changes have often resolved when positioning was altered appropriately.

Clearly, monitoring during the most critical periods of operative manipulation is useful but is not sufficient to detect even a majority of the events of interest. Continuous monitoring is optimal. Whenever possible, we prefer to institute electrophysiologic monitoring before the induction of anesthesia. Correlations between electrophysiologic measurements and clinical neurologic assessment can then be determined, and monitoring can be performed intraoperatively even if EPs are abnormal, so long as reproducible waveforms are present. Electrophysiologic monitoring is then continued until the patient is sufficiently awakened from anesthesia to permit at least a rudimentary clinical neurological examination after the operative intervention. This requires that the anesthetic be planned from the beginning to facilitate rapid, safe emergence from anesthesia, if at all possible while the patient is still in the operating room.

Quality Control in EP Monitoring

Intraoperative EP monitoring will benefit patients only if accurate recordings can be made and appropriately interpreted in the operating room.

Devices capable of recording high quality, reproducible waveforms are currently available from many manufacturers. Modern operating rooms that meet contemporary electrical safety standards usually permit satisfactory recordings on a routine basis, although filter settings may be somewhat more restrictive than those used in the diagnostic laboratory. It is very helpful to continually monitor the unprocessed EEG signal as it is acquired so that recording can be suspended when the signal is noisy. Automatic artifact rejection is quite useful, but all the currently available devices depend entirely on amplitude criteria for artifact rejection. Small signals, such as those picked up from a bipolar electrocoagulation device, are still admitted and can contaminate electrophysiologic data. Secure application of electrodes with impedances that are low and matched is crucial. Noise should be eliminated at the source, to the greatest extent possible. No amount of data processing can fully compensate for noisy recordings. Thus, EP monitoring must be performed by knowledgeable personnel to avoid technical problems that might be clinically misleading.

Interpretation of EP waveforms and appropriate use of the information provided requires the presence of a knowledgeable physician in the operating room. An individual must be present who can integrate the information from multiple monitors as well as from events in the course of anesthesia and surgery to reach meaningful conclusions about the meaning and relevance of possible changes in EPs. This person can be a neurologist, a surgeon, or an anesthesiologist. The base speciality of the individual concerned is far less important than a genuine interest in EP monitoring, a commitment to be present in the operating room, and a willingness to learn something about the other related disciplines. Postoperative interpretation of EPs does not allow for intraoperative intervention on the basis of EP findings.

Criteria for Use of Intraoperative EP Monitoring

Intraoperative EP monitoring is most likely to be appropriate when four conditions are met[8]. First, a pathway amenable to monitoring should be at risk. Second, sites must be available for stimulation and recording. Third, appropriate equipment and qualified personnel must be available to record and interpret EPs in the operating room. Finally, if the monitoring is to be of more than academic interest, there should be some possibility of intervening to improve function if EPs deteriorate or are lost.

Assessing Evoked Potentials for Intraoperative Monitoring

When new monitoring techniques are introduced for use in the operating room, the anesthesiologist and surgeon would like to know how well these techniques perform in terms of feasibility, sensitivity, utility, and reliability.

Since experiments to test performance of EP monitors cannot be carried to their logical conclusions in patients, we first carry out studies in animals. Then we must devise indicators to characterize performance of new monitoring techniques in the clinical arena[9].

The *feasibility* of intraoperative EP monitoring can be assessed by examining the availability of appropriate equipment and qualified personnel, the time requirements for monitoring in a busy operating room suite, the frequency and magnitude of technical impediments to monitoring, and the constraints, if any, that are placed on anesthetic and surgical management to facilitate monitoring. *Sensitivity* of EP monitoring techniques can be examined by carefully observing EP changes that occur in the operating room to determine their frequency and their association with events of clinical interest, such as distraction of the spine, occlusion of critical blood vessels, or placement of retractors on the brain. As reasonable indicators of *utility*, we can examine the occasions when EP data aid clinical decision making or lead to therapeutic intervention. Finally, the *reliability* of EP monitoring can be evaluated by determining the relationships between results of intraoperative monitoring and neurologic outcomes. Even though we continually strive to optimize function, not waiting for signals that would assure a bad outcome, a few patients suffer neurologic damage intraoperatively despite our best efforts. It is important to characterize the EP data recorded intraoperatively from these unfortunate individuals as completely as possible. Similarly, it is important to document the range of EP changes consistent with good outcomes. Monitoring can then be improved by better definition of safe ranges for intraoperative EP measurements.

Numerous investigators have now demonstrated that intraoperative monitoring is feasible, sensitive, useful and reliable in many applications. Problems with feasibility are diminishing with the development of better equipment and greater availability of knowledgeable personnel. As our collective clinical experience grows, both sensitivity and utility are enhanced. Problems with reliability often seem due to errors in recording or interpretation. The problems of so-called "false positives" and "false negatives" are discussed below.

Factors Affecting EPs During Anesthesia and Surgery

Many factors other than surgical intervention can affect EPs. These include body temperature, arterial blood pressure, arterial blood gas tensions, anesthetics, and stimulus and recording parameters. Many of these effects have been fully or partly characterized, but we do not have sufficient information to apply standardized correction factors to an isolated waveform from an individual patient. Little work has been done to examine the interactions among these factors[10], and almost nothing has been done to examine the interactions between these factors and abnormalities of waveforms due to preoperative pathology that affects EPs.

The important steps in minimizing these difficulties when monitoring EPs in the operating room are the following: First, preoperative recordings should be obtained before the induction of anesthesia. Even abnormal waveforms can be effectively monitored if they are reproducible and subsequent alterations are observed in relationship to clinical events of interest. Second, the monitoring team should be aware of the current state of the art with regard to signal acquisition, processing, and interpretation in the clinical setting and patient population of interest. Third, the anesthesiologist should attempt to use anesthetic techniques that facilitate both monitoring and early awakening from anesthesia, maintaining a steady state both pharmacologically and physiologically during critical steps of the surgical procedure such as distraction of the spine or occlusion of the carotid artery. Fourth, an attempt should be made to monitor a pathway not at risk from the surgical procedure. This helps to distinguish anesthetic or other systemic changes in EPs from those related to the operation. For example, we monitor SEPs from at least one median nerve as well as those from each posterior tibial nerve during operations on the thoracic or lumbar spine. Finally, communication among the monitoring personnel, the anesthesiologist, and the surgeon is vital. Active cooperation from the entire operating room team is the key to success.

Avoiding "False Positives" and "False Negatives"

Numerous reports of so-called "false positive" and "false negative" results of intraoperative EP monitoring have appeared in the literature. Most of these can be attributed to either a failure to observe the criteria for monitoring mentioned above or to a misunderstanding of the pathophysiology in a given situation. We have recently completed a detailed analysis of several such cases[11]. Problems arose when the pathway at risk was not monitored, as when only BAEPs were monitored and the cerebral cortex was injured or when the thoracic or lower cervical cord was injured but only median nerve evoked potentials were recorded. On other occasions the EPs were normal intraoperatively and the patient awoke neurologically normal but developed a deficit hours or days later (while not being monitored). In some reports either the EP waveforms or the relevant aspects of pathophysiology appear to have been misinterpreted. For example, transient loss of the BAEP due to retraction of the eighth cranial nerve for more than 100 minutes is consistent with preservation of hearing[12], while loss of the SEP during aortic surgery for longer than about 15 minutes may be associated with recovery of SEPs and dorsal column function while motor function is lost[13]. Simultaneous stimulation at more than one site may also produce confusion. Although bilateral posterior tibial nerve stimulation produces larger waveforms, a unilateral insult to the spinal cord may be missed. A case at our institution demonstrated unilateral loss of the SEP and had pathologically confirmed injury to one side of the spinal cord[14]. We use bilateral stimulation only when we are otherwise unable to elicit SEPs adequate for monitoring.

Conclusions

SEPs and BAEPs are well established as important monitors of central nervous system function in the operating room. The potential barriers to successful monitoring have been defined and are amenable to solution using presently available equipment and techniques. Many excellent examples of important clinical work are presented in the report of this symposium.

References

1. Beecher HK (1940) The first anesthesia records (Codman, Cushing). Surg Gynecol Obstet 71: 689
2. Bendixen HH (1978) A forward: the tasks of the anesthesiologist. In: Saidman LJ, Smith NT (eds) Monitoring in anesthesia. Wiley, New York, pp 227–267
3. MacEwen GD, Bunnell WP, Sriram K (1975) Acute neurological complications in the treatment of scoliosis: a report of the Scoliosis Research Society. J Bone Joint Surg 57 A: 404
4. Steed DL, Peitzmann AB, Grundy BL et al (1982) Causes of stroke in carotid endarterectomy. Surgery 92: 634
5. Grundy BL, Lina A, Procopio PT, Jannetta PJ (1981) Reversible evoked potential changes with retraction of the eighth cranial nerve. Anesth Analg 60: 835
6. Grundy BL, Jannetta PJ, Procopio PT et al (1982) Intraoperative monitoring of brain-stem auditory evoked potentials. J Neurosurg 57: 674
7. Mahla ME, Long DM, McKennett J, Green C et al (1984) Detection of brachial plexus dysfunction by somatosensory evoked potential monitoring – A report of two cases. Anesthesiology 60: 248
8. Grundy BL (1982) Monitoring of sensory evoked potentials during neurosurgical operations: methods and applications. Neurosurgery 11: 556
9. Grundy BL (1983) Intraoperative monitoring of sensory evoked potentials. Anesthesiology: 58: 72
10. Gravenstein MA, Sasse F, Hogan K (1984) Effects of stimulus rate and halothane dose on canine far-field evoked potentials. Anesthesiology 61: A 342
11. Friedman WA, Grundy BL (1987) Monitoring of sensory evoked potentials is highly reliable and helpful in the operating room. J Clin Monit 3: 38

12. Grundy BL, Procopio PT, Jannetta PJ *et al* (1982) Evoked potential changes produced by positioning for retromastoid craniectomy. Neurosurgery 10: 766
13. Kaplan BJ, Friedman WA, Alexander JA, Hampson SR (1986) Somatosensory evoked potential monitoring of spinal cord ischemia during aortic operations. Neurosurgery 19: 82

History of Evoked Potential Recording in Humans

C. A. Pagni, M. Naddeo, C. Mascari

2nd Chair of Neurosurgery, University of Torino (Italy)

In 1875 Richard Caton at the Royal Infirmary School of Medicine in Liverpool, while searching for the cerebral counterpart of du Bois-Reymond's action potential in nerve, not only found it, but, recording bipolarly with a Thomson's galvanometer from cerebral cortex in animals, noticed that there was a continuous waxing and waning of cerebral potentials[19]. Superimposed on those waves Caton found potential swings related to sensory stimulation and realized that these were a sign of impulses reaching the brain from the periphery. In the following years, he was able to find responses to stimulation of limbs and to light stimulation. After Caton, Beck[5] in Cracow, and Danilewsky[28] and Larionov[61] in St. Petersburg were successful in recording potential related to light and sound. Because they had no cameras, their findings were presented by verbal descriptions or as sketches. Thus, the potentials evoked by peripheral stimulation had already been discovered when the first pictures of cortical activity and sensory evoked potentials in animals were published by Neminsky in 1913 (Fig. 1). Detailed information on those early workers can be found in Rusinov and Rabinovich[82], and in Brazier[12, 13].

A complex evoked field potential was recorded from the surface of the spinal cord of animals for the first time by Gasser and Graham in 1933[42].

Hans Berger in 1929 was the first to record brain potentials through the unopened skull in man; thus, he was the founder of clinical electroencephalography. He demonstrated that human brain potentials were affected

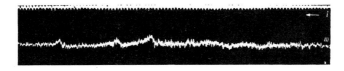

Fig. 1. The first published photograph of an evoked potential (Pravdich-Neminsky 1913)

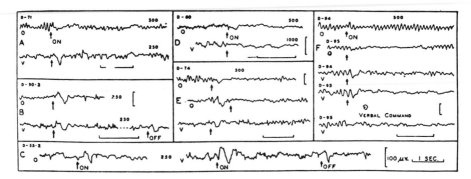

Fig. 2. The first photographs of evoked potentials in man. On-effects and modifications of spontaneous rhythms in response to sounds (P. A. Davis 1939)

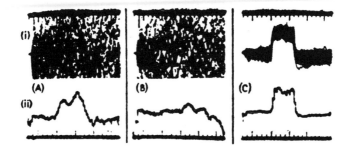

Fig. 3. A summation technique for detecting small signals. Ulnar nerve stimulation
at the wrist. The upper line of traces shows sets of 55 records superimposed; the
lower line shows the averages of these given by the machine (Dawson 1951)

by hypoxia, anesthesia, opening and closing the eyes, and sleep. He also
showed that brain waves were abnormal in epilepsy.

The first recording of a cortical evoked response to peripheral stimulation in man was published by Pauline Davis in 1939[30, 31] (Fig. 2). As her
husband Hallowel Davis wrote in 1979, evoked potentials were recorded
by Pauline following electric shocks to ring finger, flashes of light, and
sounds. However, even these were isolated observations[29].

The modern era of evoked potential recording in man was opened by
Dawson[32]. In 1947 he succeeded in recording transcranially the cerebral
responses to electrical stimulation of peripheral nerves in man by the superimposition technique. Results at the beginning were rather crude, but
in the following years he developed a new method, the "summation technique"[33], which used a rotating device synchronized with the stimulus.
With repetition of the stimulus a series of responses were led into con-
densers, each for a different time interval from the stimulus. These dis-

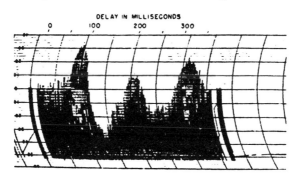

DELAY IN MILLISECONDS

0   100   200   300

Fig. 4. Cortical response in man to repeated flash. Example recorded by evoked response detector of Barlow and Brown (Barlow and Brown 1955)

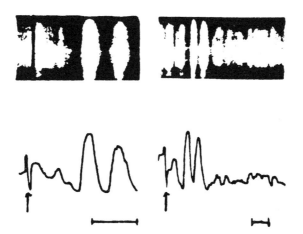

Fig. 5. The cerebral potential variations evoked by peripheral sensory stimuli are transformed in a variation of the luminosity of the beam of the cathodic oscilloscope (Calvet and Scherrer 1955)

charged in sequence, each with its proper delay in time. When recorded together these gave a summation and by scaling down appropriately a graphic average could be recorded (Fig. 3). A similar technique was employed by Barlow and Brown in 1955[4]; the pen excursion in the write-out was proportional to the voltage at that interval from the stimulus (Fig. 4).

At the same time Calvet and Sherrer[17] in France developed another recording method. The cerebral potential variations evoked by peripheral sensory stimuli were transformed in a variation − increase or decrease according to polarity − of the luminosity of the beam of the cathodic oscilloscope. The variations in potential followed at a rather constant interval the peripheral stimulus, which was synchronized with the start of the cathodic beam. Thus, the variations of luminosity were always located at the same point of the cathodic sweep. Repeated pictures of the cathodic screen were taken and superimposed on the same film, giving rise to a direct photographic integration. The photographic record was read by a photoelectric cell, producing a classical recording of potential variation (Fig. 5).

In 1956 Rémond obtained very good results with his "Phasotron," a computer-operated display which, at selected times after the stimulus, allowed the opening of gates and integrated the voltage of bioelectrical activity entering through the gates. In this way, he collected information about amplitude, polarity, and spatial distribution of the electroencephalographic variations of potentials[80].

The fundamental step for research on the evoked potentials recorded transcranially in the human, however, was the development of the first digital computing system by Clark in the Research Laboratory of Electronics at the Massachusetts Institute of Technology[21, 22]. The Average Responses Computer (A.R.C.) of Clark was the ancestor of those used today. Brazier[10] was the first to clinically employ the A.R.C. to extract evoked potentials from EEG activity recorded on the scalp (Figs. 6 and 7).

Thereafter other averaging systems were made commercially available (ERA, CAT 400 A-B-1024, ART 1000, Enhancetron).

Since then an enormous amount of clinical work has been done for both diagnostic purposes and applied physiological research. The monumental monography published in the Annals of the New York Academy of Science in 1964 is a milestone in the understanding of evoked potentials recorded in humans. Many other books that have collected growing knowledge have since been published[6, 35, 20].

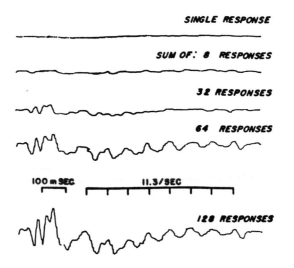

Fig. 6. Detection of evoked response to flash in man by addition of single response (ARCH-1) (Brazier 1960)

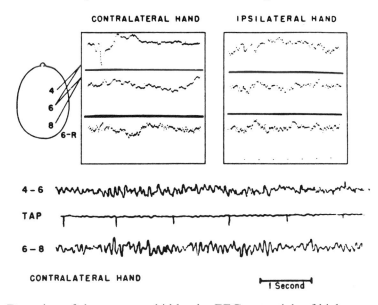

Fig. 7. Detection of the response, hidden by EEG potentials of higher amplitude, to tapping of the hand. The upper records are from the computer TX-O and show a clear evoked response at scalp electrode 4 on the contralateral hemisphere with a smaller response ipsilaterally (Brazier 1960)

Gasser and Graham[42] first described the spinal cord field potential arising from cat spinal cord after posterior root stimulation. These potentials have since been termed "cord dorsum potentials" or "intermediary cord potentials."

The first successful recordings of spinal cord potentials in man was performed by Magladery et al.[64]. The workers inserted a needle electrode into the subdural space. This technique (used also by Ertekim and Caccia in 1976[16, 37]) was associated with complications that included pain, headache, and hyperthermia; the complications were not counterbalanced by better recordings.

An alternative and less invasive method was described by Shimoji[83] who inserted a flexible copper loop into the epidural space through a Tuohy needle (Fig. 8). In 1975 Tsuyama et al. used a similar method but employed radiological control of the electrode's position[91].

A noninvasive technique using superficial skin electrodes was attempted by Liberson and Kim[63] with good results. The technique was developed and refined by Cracco[24, 25, 26] using simpler silver cups (Fig. 9). The method was subsequently employed by Jones and Small[58]. Dimitrjievic and Delbeke in 1978 used 50 × 60 mm silver strips covered by conductive paste and applied to the skin at the level of the examined spinous process. Evoked

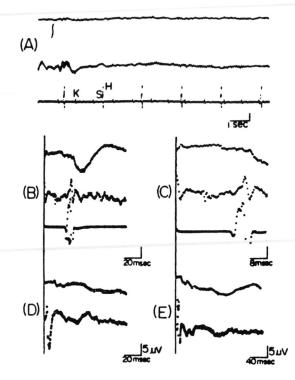

Fig. 8. Evoked spinal cord potentials by Shimoji who inserted a flexible copper loop into the epidural space through a Tuohy needle (Shimoji *et al.* 1971)

spinal cord potentials recorded noninvasively appear to be similar to those directly recorded from the spinal cord, although they are much smaller and less detailed[38].

In 1964 Brazier[12] made important contributions to the study of connections between hyppocampus, amygdala and temporal cortex in man by means of evoked response recordings. This study was done in patients with temporal lobe epilepsy who were resistant to medical therapy. Electrodes were implanted in cortical and subcortical structures for diagnostic and therapeutic purposes. The same electrodes were used for stimulation and recording.

Meanwhile, the study of evoked potentials in humans was approached in different ways and with different purposes. Neurosurgeons and neurophysiologists started to record evoked potentials directly from the brain, beginning in the late 1940s with the pioneer works of Woolsey and Walker[97], Gastaut[43], Woolsey and Erichson[95]. This work was furthered by the introduction of stereotactic techniques in neurosurgery by Spiegel and Wycis[85] (Fig. 10).

One of the main purposes in recording evoked potentials from the brain

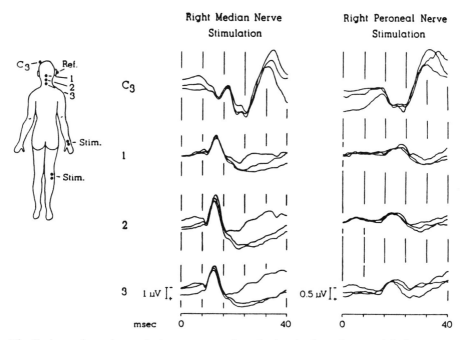

Fig. 9. A noninvasive technique to record evoked spinal cord potentials by means of superficial skin electrodes using simple silver cups (R. Q. Cracco 1973)

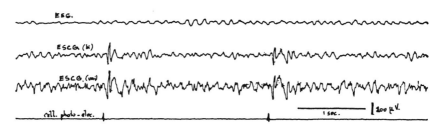

Fig. 10. Electrophysiological characteristics of subcortical evoked response recorded by Gastaut (Gastaut 1949)

was to achieve better localization of primary sensory areas during surgical exposures for resection of cerebral cortex in cases of intractable epilepsy or pain. The unique neurophysiological method for cortical localization in man was the electrical stimulation of the cerebral cortex in conscious patients. Woolsey, Walker and Erickson[97], Woolsey and Erickson[96], Pertuiset et al.[78], Hirsch et al.[53], Jasper et al.[57], and Woolsey et al.[96] attempted a correlation between the results of cortical stimulation and sensory evoked potentials recorded in conscious patients. The evoked responses to sensory peripheral stimulation were recorded from the centroparietal cortex directly

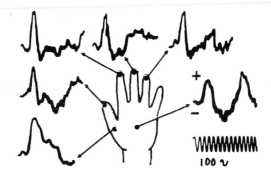

Fig. 11. Cathode ray oscillograms of evoked potentials recorded from the postcentral hand area in response to mechanical stimulation at six different loci (Walker and Woolsey 1949)

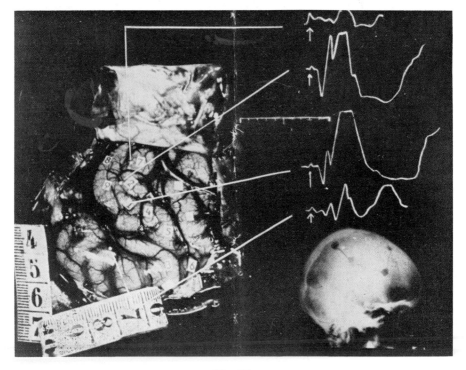

Fig. 12

Figs. 12–13. Correlation between the results of cortical stimulation and sensory evoked responses recorded in conscious patients directly on cathode-ray oscilloscope (Pertuiset *et al.* 1957, Hirsch *et al.* 1961)

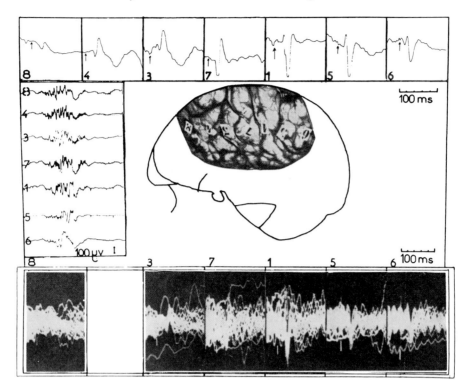

Fig. 13

on a cathode ray oscilloscope (Figs. 11–13). Jasper *et al.*[57] employed a special apparatus with a four-beam oscilloscope and a switch to select rapidly successive sets of four recording electrodes (Fig. 14).

Results of these studies may be summarized as follows:

– Evoked potentials are easily seen in single trace oscillographs by recording from cortical areas corresponding to the stimulated body region not only in conscious patients but also during general anesthesia.

– The cortical localization of sensory areas by the evoked potentials method bears a close correspondence to the localization of the same sensory areas obtained in conscious human subjects by local electrical stimulation. In fact, the initial rapid evoked potential ("primary complex") is highly stable in amplitude and location in patients with or without anesthesia and is restricted to the cortical areas whose stimulation gives rise to sensations referred to the stimulated contralateral part of the body[57, 54]. Thus the method is highly reliable.

– The area S 1 is localized in man on the postcentral gyrus, behind the Rolandic fissure and is somatotopically arranged; moreover it receives only contralateral afferents[53]. Some evoked responses were recorded from

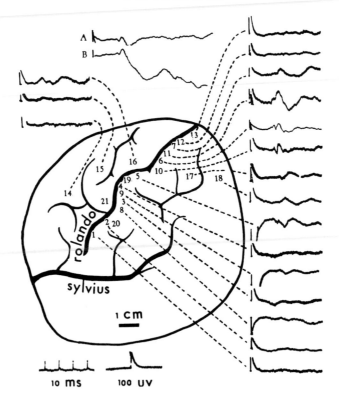

A
B

rolando

sylvius

1 cm

10 ms   100 UV

Fig. 14. Evoked responses to sensory peripheral stimulation recorded from the exposed somatosensory cortex in man (Jasper *et al.* 1960)

the precentral gyrus adjacent to the postcentral area of maximum response, but they were of lower voltage and less constant[57]. The latency seemed to be the same from the precentral gyrus as from the postcentral gyrus. Thus, somatic afferents exist in the motor cortex of the human brain. Hirsch *et al.*[53] recorded responses of the same latency but of different shape up to 3–4 cm behind the Rolandic sulcus in the parietal cortex.

In 1961, Hirsch *et al.* recorded visual evoked potentials on the external and internal surfaces of the occipital lobe. Amplitudes were greatest over the calcarine fissure. An attempt to localize the structures belonging to the primary visual pathways (geniculocortical radiations, pericalcarine cortex, fusiform lobule) was undertaken by Szikla *et al.*[88] during stereotactic exploration for focal epilepsy. Responses evoked by light flashes of short duration and recorded from the visual pathways on a cathode ray oscilloscope closely resembled the primary responses recorded during studies in animals. Latencies ranged from 30 to 50 milliseconds, depending on the point explored. The localization of responses corresponded fairly well to

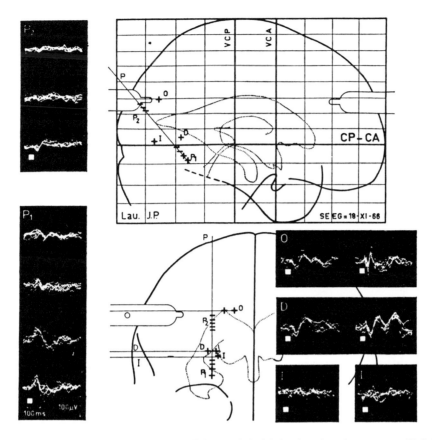

Fig. 15. Example of an exploration of the occipital lobe for visual responses (Szikla *et al.* 1967)

radiological concepts of anatomy[88] (Fig. 15). Modifications of these primary responses were observed due to changes in the physiological condition of the subject (direction of attention, opening and closing of the eyes and other stimulations)[59, 53, 73, 88]. Primary visual responses do not undergo "habituation" phenomena[72].

Visual evoked responses recorded directly from the cortex are more simple than those recorded with integration methods from the scalp. However, average responses bipolarly recorded from the exposed cortex between an electrode placed on the visual area and another in front of the visual region were remarkably similar to potentials recorded from scalp electrodes having an analogous spatial arrangement[23].

Although the specific auditory receiving area of the cerebral cortex is more distant from the scalp than the primary somatosensory and visual cortical receiving areas, nonspecific auditory evoked potentials (AEPs) have

ELECTRICAL POTENTIALS IN THE AUDITORY SYSTEM

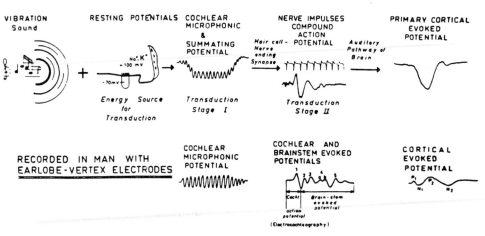

Fig. 16. Far-field recording of brainstem auditory evoked potentials (Sohmer and Feinmesser 1967)

been studied for more than 30 years. AEPs change during the various stages of natural sleep.

In 1967, Sohmer and Feinmesser[84] introduced another chapter in the history of evoked potential recording in man with far-field recording of brainstem auditory evoked potentials (BAEPs) (Fig. 16). BAEPs have largely replaced the more variable cortical AEPs for clinical neurology[86] and for the assessment of hearing in infants and other patients unable to cooperate.

Some studies suggest that sensory stimulation normally produces regional increases in local electrical activity and regional cerebral blood flow (rCBF)[39, 62]. Local cortical ischemia abolishes the cortical SEP[2, 27, 90, 50, 94].

Much physiological research has established the concept of thresholds of ischemia in the brain. Electrical function fails in progressive ischemia at levels of CBF below 18 ml/100 g/min[7, 9], while the membrane ionic pump, as indicated by the movement of potassium from intracellular to extracellular space, appears to fail only at much lower rCBF values, 9–10 ml/100 g/min[2, 8]. Such lower levels have been associated with infarction[14, 70]. It has also been shown, both experimentally and clinically[51] that, in the presence of partial loss of autoregulation characteristic of ischemic brain, induced hypertension may be employed to increase perfusion and resolve transient clinical deficits in postoperative aneurysm patients.

Changes in the brain's electrical activity can be related to CBF both experimentally and clinically. Branston *et al.*[8] demonstrated a reduction in amplitude of the trigeminal evoked potential following occlusion of the middle cerebral artery in the baboon, with a threshold relationship; the evoked potential was fully sustained down to regional blood flow levels of around 18 ml/100 g/min and substantially abolished below this level. Heiss *et al.* obtained similar results by recording unit responses in the cat[52], while Boysen and her colleagues noted in man that EEG activity disappeared at similar levels following carotid occlusion during carotid endarterectomy[7]. Subsequent increase in flow was associated with reappearance of electrical activity in several instances in both animals and humans. In an experimental model of missile injury, Crockard *et al.*[27] found that disappearance of somatosensory evoked potentials (SEPs) following median nerve stimulation was associated with rCBF below 15–20 ml/100 g/min.

SEP latency is prolonged by reduction in rCBF following MCA occlusion in the baboon[9].

Hume *et al.*[56] felt that ischemia was responsible for the prolonged central conduction time (CCT) seen in two of their nontrauma patients; this is consistent with the demonstration by Noël and Desmedt[71] that vascular lesions of the brainstem can delay the cerebral SEP. Symon *et al.* in 1979[90] suggested that the CCT may be a sensitive monitor for hemispheric dysfunction prior to the onset of a clinical ischemic deficit. As the systemic arterial pressure fell, CCT in the affected hemisphere became prolonged, and hemiparesis subsequently developed. As Heilbrun *et al.*[51] have shown following subarachnoid hemorrhage in man, and as Symon *et al.*[89] have demonstrated in ischemic lesions in baboons, autoregulation is impaired in the affected hemisphere following subarachnoid hemorrhage or an ischemic insult. Under these circumstances, therefore, a fall in systemic arterial blood pressure is associated with reduction in rCBF. Previous experience has shown that under these circumstances the appearance of a clinical deficit is attended by a proportional reduction in CBF. It appears clear, therefore, that changes in CCT are related to the development of ischemic complications; the data so far suggest that the prolongation of CCT often precedes the appearance of a clinical deficit.

Evoked potentials were employed in stereotactic surgery with the main purposes of exact localization of subcortical thalamic nuclei. In fact, because of variability in the dimensions of subcortical structures and distortions due to pathological processes such as atrophy, the coordinates of a target based on radiological landmarks and a stereotactic atlas are not sufficiently accurate. Depth EEG with macroelectrodes is not specific for various thalamic or other subcortical nuclei, so that the pattern of the record, in spite of some differences, usually cannot be used for localization of the target[93]. However, stereotactic surgery provided an opportunity to study the physiological properties of subcortical nuclei and their cortical correlations in the waking human brain.

The first attempts to record evoked potentials from the thalamic sensory

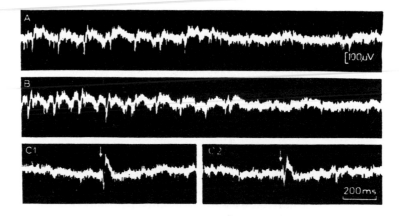

Fig. 17. Example of thalamic evoked responses recorded from the VPL nucleus
(Albe-Fessard *et al.* 1962)

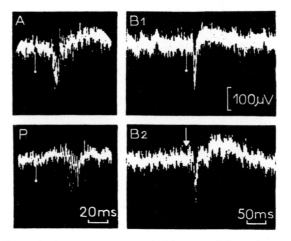

Fig. 18. Thalamic evoked responses recorded in two different patients (A and P)
and in same case (B 1—B 2) from VPL nucleus; B 1: electrical stimulation, B 2:
tactile stimulation of the index-finger (Albe-Fessard *et al.* 1962)

relay nuclei and other ascending sensory tracts at subthalamic level was
by Reyes *et al.* in 1951[81] and by Spiegel *et al.* in 1947[85]. Thereafter, the
method was successfully employed by Albe-Fessard *et al.*[1] (Figs. 17–19),
Guoit *et al.*[49], and Pagni *et al.*[75, 76].

The responses evoked in the sensory relay nuclei of the thalamus by
peripheral sensory stimulation are characterized by (a) short latency, (b)
positive initial deflection, (c) contralaterality, (d) short duration, (e) limitation to the specific projection sensory nuclei and areas, (f) striking sta-

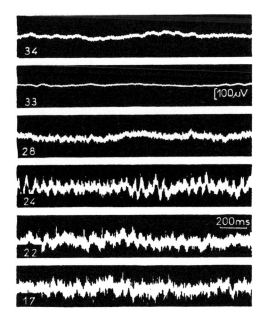

Fig. 19. Different pattern of electrical activity in thalamic nuclei and in the white matter of the internal capsule (Albe-Fessard *et al.* 1962)

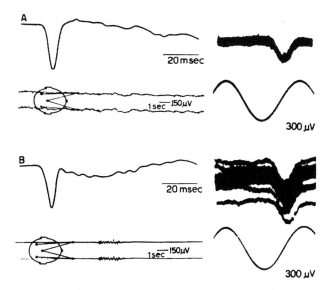

Fig. 20. Thalamic evoked responses to median nerve stimulation recorded from the VPL nucleus during thiopental anesthesia (Pagni 1967)

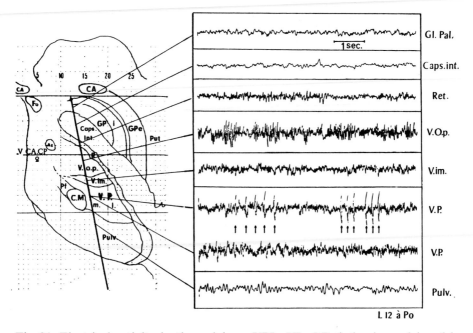

Fig. 21. Electrical activity in the pulvinar, VPL, VL, LP thalamic nuclei and in white matter of the internal capsule (Guiot *et al.* 1962)

bility during variations in attention and anesthesia[75, 76] (Fig. 20). They can probably be identified with classic "primary specific evoked responses."

Meanwhile the use of very small bipolar recording electrodes, about 20–50 microns in diameter[1], gave the opportunity to record different patterns of electrical activity in the pulvinar, VPL, VL, LP thalamic nuclei, and in the white matter of the internal capsule[49] (Fig. 21). The topographical arrangement of the sensory thalamic nuclei could be studied by recording very discrete responses evoked by peripheral stimulation. Cellular unit activity was recorded by means of microelectrodes with tips 2–3 microns in diameter[18] (Fig. 22).

These methods allowed precise recognition of the boundaries of the thalamic nuclei and identification of cellular populations and fiber bundles with different physiological functions on the basis of both spontaneous activity and potentials evoked by peripheral stimulation. The conclusion may be reached that the best method for recognizing boundaries of certain thalamic nuclei (as for instance the limit between the sensory VPL, VPM and the ventrolateral nucleus) is to use "semi-microelectrodes" 20–50 microns in diameter[1] for bipolar recording as well as evoked thalamic potentials[18].

The cortical responses evoked by stimulation of various subcortical structures were also recorded during stereotactic procedures. The "recruit-

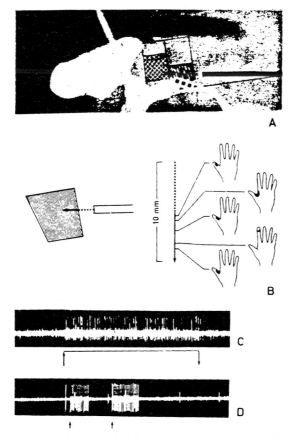

Fig. 22. Cellular unit activity recorded by means of microelectrodes (Carreras *et al.*
1967)

ing response" of Dempsey and Morison was recorded in man following
repetitive stimulation of the intralaminar thalamic nuclei[92, 55]. The stimulation of specific thalamic nuclei gave rise in man to the specific "aug-
menting responses" of Dempsey and Morison[55] (Fig. 23). Usually, however,
during stereotactic procedures in man, "mixed responses" due to the simultaneous activation of both "specific" and "nonspecific" thalamic systems were recorded from the scalp or cortex[93] (for a review see[41]). This
was perhaps due to the intensity of stimulation, duration of impulses, and
long interelectrode distances.

With extremely short (0.05 msec) rectangular impulses at threshold levels, using very short interelectrode distances, the classical primary cortical
motor response was demonstrated in man by Ganglberger *et al.*[40]. On
stimulation of the motor relay nuclei (V.o.a., V.o.p., V.o.i.), specific primary
responses with the classical surface positive-negative waveform and typical

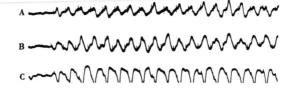

Fig. 23. Ipsilateral cortical responses registered oscillographically during the course of a single electrode placement in a 50 year old patient undergoing thalamotomy for Parkinson rigidity (Housepian and Pool 1962)

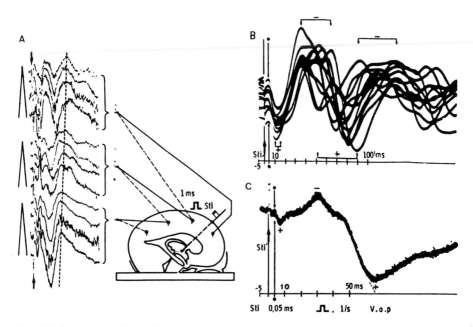

Fig. 24. On stimulation of the thalamic motor relay nuclei, specific response could be recorded from electrodes placed exactly over the related cortical projection field (Ganglberger 1982)

short latency (3–5 msec), were recorded from electrodes placed exactly over the related cortical projection field, i.e., areas 4 and 6. On increasing the stimulus intensity and/or interelectrode distance, the waveform became more complex, was followed by several slow waves (secondary responses) and spread from the motor region to the prefrontal and parietal regions.

Stimulation of the median thalamic region gives rise to cortical responses over the areas 9, 10, 11, 45, 46 and 47, similar to those elicited from motor relay nuclei but of slightly longer latency (5, 6, 7–8 msec)[41] (Fig. 24).

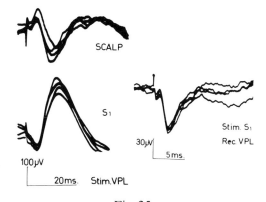

Fig. 25

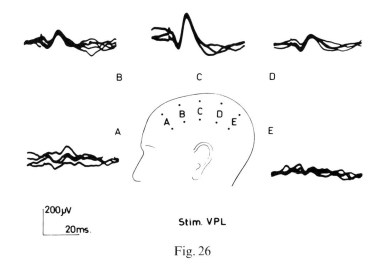

Fig. 26

Figs. 25–26. Specific primary cortical responses from the S 1 cortical area and the scalp following threshold stimulation of the specific thalamic relay nuclei (Cabrini *et al.* 1969)

Stimulation of the pulvinar gave rise to evoked responses in the ipsilateral temporoparietal and central regions, and stimulation of LP produced evoked potentials in ipsilateral frontocentral and temporal regions and in the contralateral central region.

Cabrini *et al.*[15] recorded specific primary cortical responses from the S 1 cortical area following threshold stimulation of the specific thalamic relay nuclei (VPL), by using an interelectrode distance of 4 mm and a pulse duration of 0.005–0.05 msec (Figs. 25 and 26).

The responses were recorded directly on a cathode ray oscilloscope and integrated on an Enhancetron. Latency of the response was 1.5 msec. The waveform can be exactly superimposed on the form of the specific motor response as recorded by Ganglberger[40, 41] in the area 4–6 following V.o.a.-V.o.p. stimulation. The stimulation of the recording electrode in S 1 gave a short latency response with the same latency in the VPL. With stronger stimulation of the VPL the response spread to parietal and frontal regions as could be demonstrated by scalp recording[15]. The VPL stimulation also gave rise to short latency responses in the supplementary motor area[15].

In 1964 Pagni *et al.*[73] reported observations concerning the latency and electromyographic (EMG) characteristics of motor responses obtained in man by stimulating the corticospinal tract at the capsular level. Capsular stimulation was performed during stereotactic operations using the Wyss mono- or bipolar electrode with monophasic square waves in single pulses or at frequencies of 1 to 10 Hz and pulse durations 1 to 5 msec, with intensities of 1 to 4 V. The muscular responses were recorded by surface electrodes. Stimulation of the internal capsule with single shocks evoked responses localized to the musculature of the contralateral side of the body in the form of violent muscular jerks; responses on the homolateral side of the body were never seen. The evoked motor response consisted of contraction of a single muscle or, more often, of many muscles. With stimuli of greater intensity, the responses always appeared in complex muscle systems of two limbs. Because the response generally involved agonist and

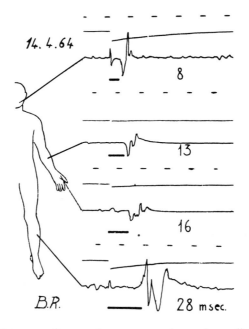

Fig. 27. Different latency of muscular response in various districts of the body following stimulation of the internal capsule (Pagni *et al.* 1964)

antagonist muscles, the amplitude of limb movements was generally small and sometimes it was very difficult to identify all the muscles involved by clinical observation. The jerks obtained in a muscle in a state of complete relaxation, using rhythmical stimuli at 1 to 4 Hz seemed, on clinical observation, to be of the same amplitude; the EMG records, on the contrary, demonstrated small, continuous variations in amplitude.

The latency between the beginning of the stimulus and the beginning of the EMG response was different for the various muscular groups and increased from head to lower limb muscles (Fig. 27; Table 1).

Table 1

Muscle or muscle group	Latency msec
M. orbicularis oris	6–9
M. deltoides	9–12
M. biceps brachii	9–15
M. extensor digitorum communis	13
M. flexores antebranchii superficiales	13
Thenar	16
M. interossei dorsales	19–20
M. quadriceps femoris	20–22
M. semitendineus et semimembranaceus	24–30
M. tibialis anterior	26–33
M. extensor digitorum brevis pedis	35

Recently a new method has been introduced to transcranially excite the motor cortex for measurements of conduction velocity in the pyramidal tract[68, 69]. Brief high-voltage electrical shocks from a special low-output resistance stimulator, delivered through electrodes on the skin, can excite muscle directly (not by way of the nerves) and can also excite the motor cortex, the visual cortex, and the spinal cord.

The first application of the new type of stimulator outside muscle was to the human motor cortex. With a pair of electrodes on the scalp, the anode over the arm area of the motor strip, twitch contractions of the opposite hand were obtained on the first attempt[68, 69]. At first these investigations used single high-voltage pulses of about 2,000 V, similar to those used on muscle but with a shorter time constant of decay (10 μs); but it was soon recognized that such high voltages are unnecessary. With fairly large stimulating electrodes (each 4 cm^2) to minimize current density at the scalp, and with pulses of 50 μs-time constant of decay, a stimulus of only a few hundred volts is required and discomfort is fully acceptable – less than when stimulating peripheral nerve for measurement of conduction velocity[67]. The stimulator must still have a low output resistance, although not so low that a stimulus transformer cannot be used to reduce shock artifact when recording electrically from muscle. A single cortical stimulus gives a synchronous muscle action potential, typically of a millivolt or a few millivolts. To the adductor of the thumb the latency is about 23 msec and to the tibialis anterior (with the stimulus to the leg area) about 34 msec. Such measurements, which are very easily made on single sweeps, will no doubt be used clinically to detect slowing of conduction in the motor pathways in demyelinating and other diseases, complementing the well established tests of conduction in the sensory pathways which use the somatosensory evoked potential.

The chief observation thought to be new here is that the threshold for cortical stimulation is much reduced if the muscle under observation makes a moderate voluntary contraction, say 20% of maximal, before stimulation[67]. This fact apparently did not emerge from observations on the brain exposed at operation or in animal experiments. It is of interest too that the excitability of the cortex, and of the whole pathway to the muscle, does not alter during the fatigue produced by 4 min of maximal voluntary contraction of the muscle; the muscle action potential caused by a cortical stimulus remains much the same[66].

In 1981 Marsden et al.[65] recorded the mechanical twitch in the adductor pollicis with the usual strain-gauge device attached to the thumb. They found unexpectedly that a single cortical stimulus not greatly above threshold voltage produced a maximal twitch in the muscle. It is perhaps surprising that all the motor neurons of the muscle should be accessible in this way to a single shock to the cortex.

Whether the same is true for muscles other than hand muscles, with their prominent cortical representation, is not yet known.

Measurement of the size of the mechanical twitch after cortical stimulus, relative to a wrist-evoked twitch, might be the basis for another quantitative test of damage to the pyramidal tract[67]. The technique of evoked potential recording from the scalp, the gasserian ganglion and root, and from peripheral trigeminal branches as the effect of pre and intraoperative stimulation of the ganglia and root has been employed both for diagnostic purposes in facial neuralgia and intraoperative monitoring of the lesion during thermal rhizotomies for typical tic douloureux (Cruccu et al. 1987 for a review).

SEPs today are useful for investigation in various branches of medicine, but in particular their use to assess neurological function in anesthetized patients is very important. Both the EEG and the cortical SEPs are altered when cerebral perfusion or oxygenation is compromised.

Although multiple-channel EEG is superior to the single-channel averaged SEP for monitoring the brain during carotid endarterectomy or cardiopulmonary bypass[45, 46, 47, 48, 87], only evoked potentials reflect the functional integrity of subcortical and cortical sensory pathways[44]. The SEPs not only reflect specific sensory transmission, but they also serve to a limited extent as more general indicators of neurological function in adjacent structures.

Several investigators have recorded SEPs during neurosurgical, orthopedic, and vascular operations that pose risks of neural injury, attempting to predict neurological outcome and minimize postoperative neurological morbidity. For instance, SEPs are monitored during operations on the spine or spinal cord, BAEPs are monitored during operations in the posterior cranial fossa, and visual evoked potentials are monitored during resection of large pituitary tumors.

Assessment of the feasibility, sensitivity, utility, and reliability of these new intraoperative monitoring methods will be discussed in the following chapters of this book.

References

1. Albe-Fessard D, Arfel G, Guiot G, Hardy J, Vuorc'h G, Hertzog E, Aleonard P, Derome P (1962) Dérivations d'activités spontanées et évoquées dans les structures cérébrales profondes de l'homme. Rev Neurol (Paris) 108: 89–105
2. Astrup J, Symon L, Branston NM, Lassen NA (1977) Cortical evoked potential and extracellular K + and H + at critical levels of brain ischemia. Stroke 8: 51–57
3. Baldissera F, Ettorre G, Infuso L, Mancia M, Pagni CA (1966) Etude comparative des réponses évoquées par stumulation des voies cortico-spinales pendant le sommeil et la veille, chez l'homme et chez l'animal. Rev Neurol 115: 82–84
4. Barlow JS, Brown RM (1955) An analog correlator system for brain potentials. Techn Rep 300. Research Laboratory of Electronics; Massachusetts Institute of Technology, Cambridge, MA, 37–39
5. Beck A (1891) Oznaczenie lokalizacyi z mòzgu i rdzeniu za pomoca zjawisk elektrycznych (Determination of localization in the brain and spinal cord by means of electrical phenomena). Presented October 20, 1890. Rozpr Wydz mat-przyr Polsk Akad Um Ser II, 1: 186–232 (doctoral thesis)
6. Bergamini G, Bergamasco B (1967) Cortical evoked potentials in man. Ch C Thomas, Springfield, Ill, pp 116
7. Boysen G, Engell HC, Trojaborg E (1973) Effect of mechanical rCBF reduction on EEG in man. Stroke 4: 361
8. Branston NM, Strong AJ, Symon L (1978) Extracellular potassium activity, evoked potentials and tissue blood flow. J Neurol Sci 45: 305–321
9. Branston NM, Symon L, Crockard A, Pazstor E (1974) Relationship between the cortical evoked potential and local cortical blood flow following acute middle cerebral artery occlusion in the baboon. Exp Neurol 45: 195–208

10. Brazier MAB (1960) Some uses of computers in experimental neurology. Exp Neurol 2: 123–140
11. Brazier MAB (1961) A history of the electrical activity of the brain: the first half-century. Pitman, London
12. Brazier MAB (1964) Evoked responses recorded from the depths of the human brain. In: Sensory evoked responses in man. Ann NY Acad Sci, Vol 112: 33–59
13. Brazier MAB (1984) Pioneers in the discovery of evoked potentials. Electroencephalogr Clin Neurophysiol 59: 2–8
14. Brierley JB, Symon L (1977) The extent of infarcts in baboon brains three years after division of the middle cerebral artery. Neuropath Appl Neurobiol 3: 217–218
15. Cabrini GP, Ettorre G, Infuso L, Marossero F, Pagni CA (1969) Studio dei potenziali corticali evocati da stimolazione del nucleo talamico VPL nell'uomo. Riv Neurol XXXIX: 12–19
16. Caccia MR, Ubiali E, Andreussi L (1976) Spinal evoked responses recorded from the epidural space in normal and diseased humans. J Neurol Neurosurg Psychiatry 39: 962–972
17. Calvet J, Scherrer J (1955) De certains possibilités et limites dans les mesures électrophysiologiques. Actes des Journées "Mesure et Connaissance". Rev Mét (Paris), pp 289–293
18. Carreras M, Pagni CA, Mancia D (1967) Unit discharges recorded from the human thalamus with microelectrodes. Confin Neurol 29: 87–89
19. Caton R (1875) The electric currents of the brain. Br Med J 2: 278
20. Chiappa HK (1983) Evoked potentials in clinical medicine. Raven Press, New York, pp 99, 340
21. Clark WA (1958) Average response computer (ARCH-1). Quart Progr Rep, Research Laboratory of Electronics, M.I.T., Cambridge MA, pp 114–117
22. Clark WA, Brown RM, Goldstein MH Jr, Molnar CE, O'Brien DF, Zieman HE (1961) The average response computer (ARC): a digital device for computing averages and amplitude and time histograms of electrophysiological response. IRE Trans Bio-med Electron 8 (BME-8): 46–51
23. Corletto F, Gentilomo A, Rosadini G, Rossi GF, Zattoni J (1966) Corrélations entre niveau de conscience, EEG et potentials évoquées chez l'homme. Rev Neurol 115: 5–14
24. Cracco RQ (1973) Spinal evoked response: Peripheral nerve stimulation in man. Electroencephalogr Clin Neurophysiol 35: 379–386
25. Cracco JB, Cracco RQ, Graziani LJ (1975) The spinal evoked response in infants and children. Neurology (NY) 25: 31–36
26. Cracco JB, Cracco RQ, Stolove R (1979) Spinal evoked potential in man: A maturational study. Electroencephalogr Clin Neurophysiol 46: 58–64
27. Crockard HA, Brown FD, Trimble J, Mullan JF (1977) Somatosensory evoked potentials, cerebral blood flow and metabolism following cerebral missile trauma in monkeys. Surg Neurol 7: 281–287
27 a. Cruccu G, Inghilleri M, Manfredi M, Heglio M (1987) Intracranial stimulation of the trigeminal nerve in man III. Sensory potentials. J Neurol Neurosurg Psychiatry 50: 1323–1330

28. Danilevsky VJ (1891) Zur Frage über die electromotorischen Vorgänge im Gehirn als Ausdruck seines Tätigkeitszustandes. Centralbl Physiol, Bd v.n. 1

29. Davis H Alfred Lee Loomis (1979) American discoverer of the EEG (personal communication). Med Coll Univ of Virginia

30. Davis PA (1939 a) Effects of acoustic stimuli on the waking human brain. J Neurophysiol 2: 494–499

31. Davis PA (1939) The electrical response of the human brain to auditory stimuli. Am J Physiol 126: 475–476

32. Dawson GD (1947) Cerebral responses to electrical stimulation of peripheral nerve in man. J Neurol Neurosurg Psychiatry 10: 134–140

33. Dawson GD (1951) A summation technique for detecting small signals in a large irregular background. J Physiol (Lond) 115: 2 P–3 P

34. Delbeke J, Mc Comas AJ, Kopec SJ (1978) Analysis of evoked lumbosacral potentials in man. J Neurol Neurosurg Psychiatry 41: 293–302

35. Desmedt JE, Noel P (1973) Average cerebral evoked potentials in the evaluation of lesions of the sensory nerves and of the central somatosensory pathways. In: Desmedt JE (ed) New developments in electromyography and clinical neurophysiology, vol 2. S Karger, Basel, pp 352–371

36. Dimitrijevic MR, Larsson LE, Lehmkuhl D, Sherwood A (1978) Evoked spinal cord and nerve root potentials in humans using a noninvasive recording technique. Electroencephalogr Clin Neurophysiol 45: 331–340

37. Ertekin C (1976) Studies on the human evoked electrospinogram. Acta Neurol Scand 53: 3–20

38. Feldman MH, Cracco RQ, Farmer P, Mount F (1980) Spinal evoked potential in the monkey. Ann Neurol 7: 238–244

39. Foit A, Larsen B, Hattori S, Skinhoj E, Lassen NA (1980) Cortical activation during somatosensory stimulation and voluntary movement in man: A regional cerebral blood flow study. Electroencephalogr Clin Neurophysiol 50: 426–436

40. Ganglberger JA, Gestring GF, Groll E, Guttmann G, Haider M (1969) Computer analysis of thalamic and cortical evoked potentials in man. Electroencephalogr Clin Neurophysiol 26: 441

41. Ganglberger JA (1982) Cortical Evoked Potentials. In: Schaltenbrand G, Walker AE (eds) Stereotaxy of the human brain. G Thieme, Stuttgart New York, pp 334–347

42. Gasser HS, Graham HT (1933) Potentials produced in the spinal cord by stimulation of dorsal roots. Am J Physiol 103: 303–320

43. Gastaut H (1949) Enregistrement sous-cortical de l'activité électrique spontanée et provoquée du lobe occipital humain. Electroencephalogr Clin Neurophysiol 1: 205–221

44. Greenberg RP, Ducker TB (1982) Evoked potentials in the clinical neurosciences. J Neurosurg 56: 1–18

45. Grundy BL, Sanderson AC, Webster MW, Richey ET, Procopio P, Karanjia PN (1981 a) Hemiparesis following carotid endarterectomy: Comparison of monitoring methods. Anesthesiology 55: 462–466

46. Grundy BL, Webster MW, Nelson P, Sanderson AC, Karanjia P, Troost BT

(1981 b) Brain monitoring during carotid endarterectomy. Anesthesiology 55 (3 A): A 129 (abstr)

47. Grundy BL (1982) Monitoring of sensory evoked potentials during neurosurgical operations: Methods and applications. Neurosurgery 11: 556–575

48. Grundy BL (1983) Intraoperative monitoring of sensory-evoked potentials. Anesthesiology 58: 72–87

49. Guiot G, Hardy J, Albe-Fessard D (1962) Délimitation précise des structures sous-cortical et identification de noyaux thalamiques chez l'homme par l'électrophysiologie stéréotaxique. Neurochirurgie 5: 1–18

50. Hargadine JR, Branston NM, Symon L (1980) Central conduction time in primate brain ischemia − a study in baboons. Stroke 11: 637–642

51. Heilbrun NP, Olsen J, Lassen NA (1972) Regional cerebral blood flow studies in subarachnoid hemorrhage. J Neurosurg 37: 36–44

52. Heis WO, Waltz AG, Hayakawa T (1975) Neuronal function and local blood flow during experimental cerebral ischemia. In: Harper AM, Jennet WB, Miller JD *et al* (eds) Blood flow and metabolism in the brain. Churchill Livingstone, Edinburgh, pp 14–27

53. Hirsch JF, Pertuiset B, Calvet J, Buisson-Ferey J, Fischgold H, Scherrer J (1961) Etude des réponses électrocorticales obtenues chez l'homme par des stimulations somesthésiques et visuelles. Electroencephalogr Clin Neurophysiol 13: 411–424

54. Hirsch JF, Buisson-Ferey J (1963) Potentiels évoqués en neurochirurgie. In: Fischgold H, Dreyfus-Brisac C, Pruvot P (eds) Problèmes de base en électroencéphalographie. Masson, Paris, pp 103–115

55. Housepian EM, Pool JL (1962) Application of stereotaxic methods to histochemical, electronmicroscopic and electrophysiological studies of human subcortical structures. Confin Neurol 22: 171–177

56. Hume AL, Cant BR (1978) Conduction time in central somatosensory pathways in man. Electroencephalogr Clin Neurophysiol 45: 361–375

57. Jasper H, Lende R, Rasmussen T (1960) Evoked potentials from the exposed somato-sensory cortex in man. J Nerv Ment Dis 130: 526–537

58. Jones SJ, Small DG (1978) Spinal and sub-cortical evoked potentials following stimulation of the posterior tibial nerve in man. Electroencephalogr Clin Neurophysiol 44: 299–306

59. Jouvet M, Cuorjon J (1958) Variations des réponses visuelles sous-corticales au cours de l'attention chez l'homme. Rev Neurol (Paris) 99: 177

60. Kano T, Shimojik (1974) The effects of ketamine and neuroleptanalgesia on the evoked electrospinogram and electromyogram in man. Anesthesiology 40: 241–246

61. Larionov VE (1897) On the cortical centers of hearing in dogs. Obozr Psychiat Neurol (St Petersburg) 2: 419–424 (in Russian)

62. Leninger-Follert E, Hossmann KA (1979) Simultaneous measurements of microflow and evoked potentials in the somatomotor cortex of the cat brain during specific sensory activation. Pfluegers Arch 380: 85–89

63. Liberson WT, Kim KC (1963) Mapping evoked potential elicited by stimulation of the median and peroneal nerves. Electroencephalogr Clin Neurophysiol 15: 721

64. Magladery JW, Porter WE, Park AM, Teasdall RD (1951) Electrophysiological studies of nerve and reflex activity in normal man, IV. The motoneurone reflex and identification of two action potentials from spinal roots and cord. Bull the Hopkins Hospital 88: 199–519

65. Marsden CD, Merton PA, Morton HB (1981) Maximal twitches from stimulation of the motor cortex in man. J Physiol 312: 5 P

66. Merton PA, Hill DK, Morton HB (1981) Indirect and direct stimulation of fatigued human muscle. In: Human muscle fatigue. Ciba Founds Symp. no 82. Pitman Medical, London, pp 120–129

67. Merton PA, Hill DK, Morton HB, Marsden CD (1982) Scope of a technique for electrical stimulation of human brain, spinal cord, and muscle. Lancet ii: 597–600

68. Merton PA, Morton HB (1980 a) Stimulation of the cerebral cortex in the intact human subject. Nature 285: 227

69. Merton PA, Morton HB (1980 b) Electrical stimulation of human motor and visual cortex through the scalp. J Physiol 305: 9–10 P

70. Morawetz R, De Girolami B, Ojemann RG, Marcoux FW, Cromwell RM (1978) Cerebral blood flow determined by hydrogen clearance during middle artery occlusion in unanaesthetised monkeys. Stroke 9: 143–149

71. Noel P, Desmedt JE (1975) Somatosensory cerebral evoked potentials after vascular lesions of the brainstem and diencephalon. Brain 98: 113–128

72. Pagni CA, Ettorre G, Marossero F, Infuso L, Cassinari V (1964 a) Primary visual potentials in man during repetitive photic stimulation. Experientia (Basel) 20: 641

73. Pagni CA, Ettorre G, Infuso L, Marossero F (1964 b) EMG responses to capsular stimulation in the human. Experientia (Basel) 20: 691

74. Pagni CA, Ettorre G, Infuso L, Marossero F, Cassinari V (1965) Risposte muscolari ottenute per stimoli capsulari nell'uomo: Latenza e caratteri elettromiografici. Boll Soc Ital Sper 46: 37–40

75. Pagni CA, Cabrini GP, Marossero F, Infuso L, Ettorre G (1966) Applicazione alla neurochirurgia sterotassica di una tecnica neurofisiologica: la registrazione dei potenziali evocati sensitivi talamici. Riv Neurol 36: 243–250

76. Pagni CA, Carreras M, Mancia D (1967) Esplorazione microfisiologica del talamo nell'uomo. Qualche osservazione sulle proprietà funzionali dei neuroni di relais somato-sensoriale. Riv Neurol 37: 441–446

77. Pagni CA (1967) Somatosensory evoked potentials in thalamus and cortex of man. In: Cobb W, Morocutti C (eds) The evoked potentials. Electroencephalogr Clin Neurophysiol [Suppl] 26: 147–155

78. Pertuiset B, Hirsch JF, Calcet J, Lefranc E (1959) Evocation corticale et souscorticale d'un membre fantome douloureux. (Stimulation et enregistrement cortical: stimulation et coagulation souscorticale.) Rev Neurol 101: 140–148

79. Pravdich-Neminsky VV (1913) Ein Versuch der Registrierung der elektrischen Gehirnerscheinungen (Experiments on the registration of the electrical phenomena of the mammalian brain). Z Physiol 27: 951–960

80. Rémond A (1956) Intégration temporelle et intégration spatiale à l'aide d'un même appareil. Rev Neurol 95: 585–586

81. Reyes V, Henny GC, Baird H, Wycis HT, Spiegel EA (1951) Localization of centripetal pathways of the human brain by recording of evoked potentials. Trans Am Neurol Assoc 76: 246–248

82. Rusinov VS, Rabinovich MY (1958) Electroencephalographic researches in the laboratories and clinics of the Soviet Union. Electroencephalogr Clin Neurophysiol [Suppl] 8: 1–36

83. Shimoji K, Hihashi H, Kano T (1971) Epidural recording of spinal electrogram in man. Electroencephalogr Clin Neurophysiol 30: 236–239

84. Sohmer H, Feinmesser M (1967) Cochlear action potentials recorded from the external ear in man. Ann Otol Rhinol Laryngol 76: 427–435

85. Spiegel EA, Wycis HT, Marks M, Lee AJ (1947) Stereotaxic apparatus for operation on the human brain. Science 106: 349–350

86. Stockard JJ, Sharbrough FW (1980) Unique contributions of short-latency auditory and somatosensory evoked potentials to neurological diagnosis. Prog Clin Neurophysiol 7: 231–263

87. Sundt TM, Sharbrough FW, Pipgras DG, Kearns TP, Messick JM, O'Fallon WM (1981) Correlation of cerebral blood flow and electroencephalographic changes during carotid endarterectomy. Mayo Clin Proc 56: 533–543

88. Szikla G, Bordas-Ferrer M, Buser P (1967) Studies on stereotaxic localization of optic radiations in man. Anatomo-radiological and physiological data. Confin Neurol 29: 175–180

89. Symon L, Branston NM, Strong AJ (1976) Autoregulation in acute focal ischemia. Stroke 7: 547–554

90. Symon L, Hargadine J, Zawirski M, Branston NM (1979) Central conduction time as a index of ischemia in subarachnoid hemorrhage. J Neurol Sci 44: 99–103

91. Tsuyama N, Tsuzuki N, Kurokawa T, Imai D (1975) Clinical applications of spinal cord action potential measurement. Hongo, Bunkyo, KU 7-3-1, 1–16

92. Umbach W (1961) Cortical responses to subcortical stimulation of the diffuse projecting system in 662 stereotaxic operations in men. Excerpta Med Int Congr Series 37: 76

93. Umbach W (1966) Elektrophysiologische und vegetative Phänomene bei stereotaktischen Hirnoperationen. Springer, Berlin Heidelberg New York, 163

94. Umbach C, Heiss WD, Traupe H (1981) Effect of graded ischemia on functional coupling and components of somatosensory evoked potentials. J Cereb Blood Flow Metab 1: 198–199 (abstr)

95. Woolsey CN, Erickson TC (1950) Study of the postcentral gyrus of man by the evoked potential technique. Trans Am Neurol Ass 75: 50–52

96. Woolsey CN, Erickson TC, Gilson WE (1979) Localization in somatic sensory and motor areas of human cerebral cortex as determined by direct recording of evoked potentials and electrical stimulation. J Neurosurg 51: 476–506

97. Woolsey CN, Walker AE, Erickson TC (1949) Somatic afferent representation in the cerebral cortex of man. International Neurological Congress, Paris

Somatosensory Evoked Potential Monitoring During Intracranial Aneurysm Surgery

R. Villani, A. Landi, A. Ducati, E. Fava*, M. Cenzato, R. Massei**

Institute of Neurosurgery and * CNR Institute for Muscle Physiology, c/o Institute of Neurosurgery, ** II Chair of Anesthesiology, University of Milano (Italy)

Introduction

Intracranial aneurysm surgery requires particular care in surgical technique, timing and pre- and postoperative management[2].

The arterial spasm and brain ischemia that follow subarachnoid hemorrhage (SAH) may compromise the results of surgical intervention. During surgery it is mandatory to avoid further focal spasm due to operative manipulation of vessels; spasm is more likely when the autoregulation has been fully or partially lost[1].

In order to minimize the risks of manipulating the aneurysm wall and make brain retraction easier, pharmacologically induced hypotension is used. The hypotension may reduce cerebral perfusion as well. It has been found that with a mean arterial pressure below 50 torr the electroencephalogram (EEG) becomes abnormal[6]. The EEG abnormality signifies a regional cerebral blood flow below 20 ml/100 g/min[5].

Vasodilator drugs commonly used to produce hypotension are trimetaphane, nitroprusside and nitroglycerin, with a preference for the latter. The reduction in brain perfusion produced by hypotension can be further worsened by increased intracranial pressure (ICP) or by impaired venous drainage.

Thus, preoperatively the brain may suffer vascular spasm due to SAH. During surgery, the brain may be injured by global hypoperfusion due to induced hypotension, by local ischemia due to brain retraction, by arterial spasm related to manipulation, or by accidental occlusion of a terminal artery, such as a perforating artery.

Intraoperative electrophysiologic monitoring, to give information about central nervous system (CNS) function, seems to be very useful. Different authors propose both EEG and evoked potentials (EP) for this goal[3, 7, 8].

In this report we describe 32 cases of intraoperative monitoring by means of somatosensory evoked potentials (SEPs) during intracranial aneurysm surgery. SEP alterations were related with anesthesiologic parameters, with surgical manoeuvres, and with the postoperative outcomes of the patients.

Methods and Materials

32 patients undergoing cerebrovascular surgery for intracranial aneurysm were studied. 18 were males and 14 were females; ages ranged from 19 to 52 years (mean 31 years).

All patients presented with a clinical history of SAH. Each was studied by means of arteriography and CT scan. The patients were clinically graded according to the Hunt and Hess scale[4]. Aneurysms showed the following distribution: 12 on the anterior communicating artery, 13 on the posterior communicating-intracranial carotid complex, and 7 on the middle cerebral artery.

The anesthetic management was as follows: Induction was accomplished by injection of sodium thiopental, 5–7 mg/kg, and succinylicholine, 1 mg/kg, and anesthesia was maintained with a mixture of N_2O and O_2 (2 : 1) and enflurane at a concentration from 0.8 to 1%. Hypotension was induced by means of an infusion of nitroglycerin at a concentration of 4 mcg/ml. Mean arterial blood pressure (MAP), electrocardiogram (ECG), heart rate and body temperature were monitored continuously, while arterial PO_2, PCO_2, pH and plasma electrolyte measurements were carried out at intervals. Esophageal temperature was in the range of 35.5–36 degrees Celsius.

Patients were positioned supine with the head rotated 30 degrees to the side. A frontotemporal bone flap was made to reach the underlying structures and self-retaining retractors were placed. Aneurysms were excluded using Sugita clips. SEPs were recorded when the patient had reached a well established anesthesia level to obtain a reference trace, using commercial systems (Amplaid MK 10 and Amplaid MK 15).

During surgery a recording was made every ten minutes and continuously during hypotension, vessel manipulation or clip positioning.

Stimulation was with square wave electrical pulses of 0.2 msec duration, 20 mA intensity, at a rate of 1 or 4 pulses per second delivered using subdermal needle electrodes placed at the median nerve at the wrist, bilaterally. This method of stimulation is preferred to surface electrodes, placed by elastic bands, because the bands may produce venous stasis.

Recordings were obtained using subdermal platinum needle electrodes placed over the 2nd cervical spinous process (SC 2) (+) and on C 3' and C 4' (+) referenced to FpZ (−). A ground electrode was placed on the arm. Recordings were obtained averaging 500 traces using an automatic artifact suppression system. Filtering bandwidths were, respectively, 10 to 2500 Hz for short latency SEPs (SSEPs) and 1 to 100 Hz for cortical SEPs (CSEPs). Analysis times were 30 msec for SSEPs and 200 msec for CSEPs. We evaluated the SC 2—C 3′ or C 4′ interpeak latency, the so called central conduction time (CCT) and the amplitude and morphology of cortical traces (CSEPs).

Each recording was assessed with reference to MAP values and surgical events.

Results

Preoperative clinical evaluation of the 32 patients, according to the Hunt and Hess scale, showed that 3 patients were grade 0, 19 were grade I, 6 were grade II and 4 were grade III. No patient grade 0 or I had a preoperative prolongation of the CCT either unilaterally or bilaterally, while all patients grade II and III had an unilateral or bilateral prolongation of the CCT (unilateral in 6 and bilateral in 4).

Hypotension always caused marked changes of SEPs in terms of CCT prolongation and decreased amplitudes of late waves. These changes were exacerbated by excessive retraction on the brain. When this happens, it is mandatory to remove the retractor, to proceed to further removal of cerebrospinal fluid, and to place the retractor more gently.

The extent of SEP changes in patients with good postoperative outcomes differed from that of those patients with poor outcome.

The 26 patients who did not show postoperative deterioration (all those with grade 0 or I and 4 of those with grade II) never exhibited an intraoperative prolongation of CCT exceeding 2.4 msec. The maximum absolute value of CCT in this group was 8.7 msec. Moreover, their late waves, although decreased during deliberate hypotension, were always recognizable. Late waves were diminished when the mean arterial pressure was decreased to a value of 60 torr during aneurysm dissection and clipping; this time averaged 27 minutes, ranging from 18 to 42 minutes (Fig. 1). The SEP changes partially recovered when the pressure was increased again, but in 14 cases a significant prolongation of the central conduction time (up to 1.3 msec) and a reduction of late waves, as compared to baseline recordings, were still present at the end of the surgery.

The remaining 6 patients, who had poor postoperative outcomes, showed intraoperative CCT prolongation that always reached or exceeded 9.5 msec. In this group of patients, the CCT changes appeared when the mean arterial blood pressure was decreased to the level of 75 torr (Fig. 2) for 30–95 minutes. Moreover, at this level of MAP, the amplitude of the SEP initial cortical positivity decreased and the late waves disappeared. When the MAP was further decreased to 60 torr for aneurysm clipping, the SEP changes were exacerbated.

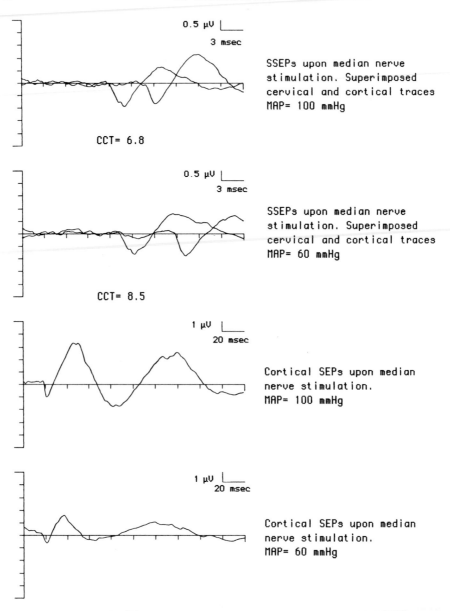

Fig. 1. Patient C. F. (anterior communicating artery aneurysm): SSEPs (upper traces – cervical and cortical traces superimposed) and cortical SEPs upon median nerve stimulation in a patient not deteriorated after surgery. The preoperative CCT was normal (6.2 msec) and symmetrical. The intraoperative CCT, on the side of the surgical approach, at a MAP of 100 mmHg, is at the upper limits of normal; on the other side it is 6.5. The same interhemispheric difference persists when the CCT increases upon decreasing the MAP to 60 mmHg. Negativity downward

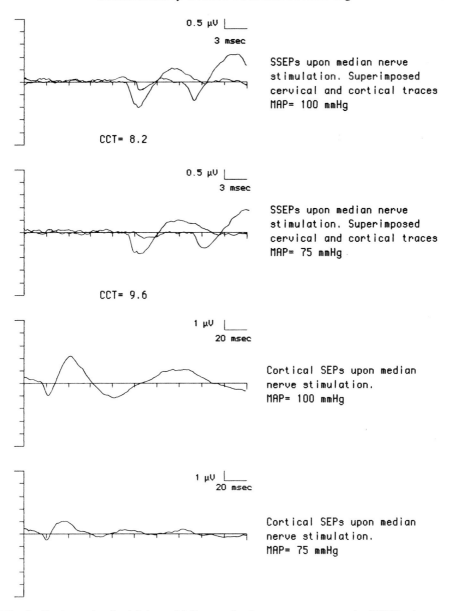

Fig. 2. Patient A. S. (right middle cerebral artery aneurysm): SSEPs (upper traces – cervical and cortical traces superimposed) and CSEPs upon left median nerve stimulation in a patient deteriorated after surgery. The preoperative right CCT was abnormal (7.7 msec); the left one was within normal limits (6.4 msec). There is a marked interhemispheric difference of CCT during surgery, at any level of MAP (left CCT 7.6 and 8.7 msec for MAP 100 and 75 mmHg respectively). CSEPs show abnormal amplitudes of late waves at the beginning of surgery, and disappearance, associated with a reduction of primary component as well, upon decreasing the MAP to 75 mmHg. Negativity downward

Of these 6 unfortunate patients, 2 died and 4 showed motor disabilities. The 2 patients who died had bilateral intraoperative prolongation of the CCT above 9.5 msec, with amplitude reduction of the initial cortical SEP to less than 50% of baseline values. The other 4 patients had predominantly unilateral alterations and, after surgery, they had severe motor impairments. The most severe and persistent disabilities were observed in the 2 patients showing unilateral intraoperative disappearance of cortical responses for more than 10 minutes.

Discussion

In our series, all the patients showed remarkable SEP alterations during aneurysm surgery, as a consequence of deliberate hypotension or brain retraction.

Patients grade II and III according to the Hunt and Hess scale showed SEP derangements before surgery that may have been due to vascular spasm following the SAH. These patients present with a damaged cerebral tissue and they are at particular risk for surgery; as a consequence, tolerance limits for SEP derangements are much more narrow for these patients than for patients grade 0 or I. We observed that an absolute CCT greater than 9.5 msec was associated with a poor postoperative outcome. Preoperative SEP recordings are necessary to assess the risk of anesthesia and surgery.

The duration of induced hypotension appears to be a critical factor. We noted that significant but short-lasting SEP alterations due to hypotension may be substantially restored within the time of surgery and are then not associated with postoperative worsening of the neurological status. On the other hand, long-lasting SEP alterations due to prolonged hypotension did not fully recover and were reliable predictors of postoperative complications.

SEPs are very sensitive neurophysiological indicators of ischemic cerebral damages. Rosenstein *et al.*[5] demonstrated that when the mean hemispheric blood flow falls below 30 ml/100 g/min the somatosensory responses show significant abnormalities in humans. All our patients seem to have reached or exceeded this value. This is potentially dangerous for the brain. According to our experience, no postoperative worsening is however to be expected when the central conduction time does not exceed 8.7 msec and when this level of SEP change persists no longer than 42 minutes. These values are obviously reached and exceeded more easily by patients whose preoperative CCT is already prolonged as a consequence of an ischemic brain insult. Moreover, a minor reduction of blood flow is sufficient to critically decrease the cerebral perfusion; when hypotension is required the SEP alterations last longer.

In conclusion, the clinically acceptable limits of SEP change are to be described not only in terms of intraoperative prolongation, but also in terms of the absolute values of central conduction time that must not be exceeded and in terms of the temporal duration of these SEP changes.

References

1. Allcock JM, Drake CG (1965) Ruptured intracranial aneurysms: the role of arterial spasm. J Neurosurg 22: 21–29
2. Drake CG (1976) Cerebral aneurysm surgery: an update. Princeton Conference, Jan
3. Eisemberg HM, Turner JW, Teasdale G (1979) Monitoring of cortical excitability during induced hypotension in aneurysm surgery. J Neurosurg 50: 595–602
4. Hunt WE, Hess RM (1968) Surgical risk related to time of intervention in the repair of intracranial aneurysms. J Neurosurg 28: 14–20
5. Rosenstein J, Wang ADJ, Symon L, Suzuki M (1985) Relationship between hemispheric cerebral blood flow, central conduction time and clinical grade in aneurysmal subarachnoid hemorrhage. J Neurosurg 62: 25–30
6. Sironi VA, Ravagnati L, Signoroni G (1982) Analisi spettrale dell'EEG durante interventi chirurgici per aneurismi cerebrali in ipotensione controllata. Riv Ital di EEG e Neurofisiol Clinica 5: 109
7. Symon L, Wang ADJ (1984) Perioperative use of somatosensory evoked responses in aneurysmal surgery. J Neurosurg 60: 269–275
8. Wang ADJ, Cone J, Symon L (1984) Somatosensory evoked potentials monitoring during the management of aneurysmal SAH. J Neurosurg 60: 264–268

Normal and Pathologic Factors Affecting Sensory Tract Potentials in the Human Spinal Cord During Surgery

S. J. JONES

Medical Research Council, National Hospital for Nervous Diseases, London
(England)

Many studies have described the morphology and properties of somato-sensory evoked potentials (SEPs) generated in the peripheral nerves, spinal cord and cerebral hemispheres in man, and a variety of techniques are now employed for monitoring the sensory pathways during surgery. The following is a survey of the major factors, technical, physiologic and pathologic, which influence afferent fiber tract potentials originating in the spinal cord. A better understanding of these will assist us in choosing appropriate recording parameters for specific applications, will help us comprehend the significance of deteriorating and abnormal records, and may provide us with insights into the physiological conduction characteristics of the normal human spinal cord.

Technical Factors

Recording Electrode Configuration

Whether recorded from the skin, bone, epidural space or pial surface, SEPs can only be detected by a pair of electrodes attached at differently influenced locations on the body. If the location of the "reference" electrode can be assumed to be largely indifferent to the evoked activity, the changes in potential at the "active" site will be displayed in undistorted form, thereby constituting a "monopolar" record. In many circumstances it is debatable whether a truly monopolar configuration can ever be achieved, but recordings obtained from sites in close proximity to the cord (the pial surface or epidural space) with reference to a more remote site such as the paraspinal muscles are essentially monopolar in character. Of course, spinal SEPs can also be recorded bipolarly, with an electrode pair laid longitudinally over the cord[5]. This has the advantage of reducing the level of background "noise" which, if present equally at the two electrodes, will be cancelled by the process of differential amplification. A disadvantage of bipolar recordings, however, is that it may no longer be possible to ascribe an individual peak in the recorded waveform to the activity of a single fiber group or tract. Close spacing of bipolar electrodes will result in a reduction in the amplitude of the recorded potential, but a wider spacing of approximately 5 cm will actually tend to enhance the amplitude of peaks recorded epidurally from the upper thoracic or lower cervical region.

Recording Frequency Bandwidth

The energy contained in spinal SEPs recorded epidurally lies very largely within the frequency band 100 Hz to 2 KHz. Consequently, the amplifier low-frequency roll-off (typically 6 dB or 50% attenuation per octave) may start as high as 200 Hz without causing major distortion of the waveform. This has the advantage that up to 75% of the main frequency (50 or 60 Hz) noise will be excluded. High-frequency filtration has little effect on the major spinal SEP components with the roll-off commencing at 1 KHz but may result in significant distortion of the waveform at a setting of 500 Hz.

Proximity of Recording Electrodes

Obviously, spinal SEPs are the best recorded when the electrode is in close proximity to the cord, but in most (particularly orthopedic) surgical applications direct contact with the pial surface is not desirable. There is also the disadvantage that the "field of view" of the electrode may be limited

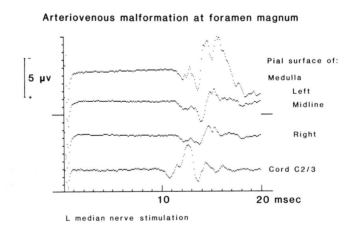

Fig. 1. Recordings obtained from the pial surface of the left, midline and right medulla and the dorsum of the spinal cord at C 2/3, following left median nerve stimulation at the wrist, illustrating the mainly ipsilateral projection at the medullary level

to a subsection of the cord, so that a defect confined to another sector might be missed. On the other hand, by using pial surface electrodes it can easily be demonstrated that the majority of activity recorded at spinal or medullary level arises in tracts ascending ipsilateral to the stimulated limb (Fig. 1), and that some components are more lateralized than others.

For an electrode in the dorsal epidural space the lateral field of view is wider, although the recorded amplitude is still considerably larger if placement is towards the ipsilateral side. Fluctuations in amplitude of up to 50% occurring during surgery may be accounted for, at least in part, by shifts in the position of the electrode tip, particularly when there has been manipulation of the vertebral column.

Increasing the separation of the electrode from the cord also increases its longitudinal field of view. This has a "smoothing" effect on the waveform, resulting in a loss of high-frequency detail and a reduction of amplitude. Smoothing is naturally more pronounced when the electrode is attached to the vertebral bone or skin, and in the latter case results in a loss of information comparable to the effect of high-frequency filtration at 500 Hz or less. It follows that there is little point in using the skin-surface waveform to investigate more fundamental aspects of spinal cord conduction.

Physiologic Factors

Fibers Activated

It may safely be assumed that per- or transcutaneous electrical stimulation of a mixed nerve with an intensity sufficient to produce a brisk but submaximal contraction of the innervated muscles will activate the majority of large diameter (Groups I and II) sensory fibers present but leave the small myelinated and unmyelinated axons quiescent. Differences in the waveform and conduction velocity of potentials recorded from the cord following stimulation of different nerves will therefore reflect differences in the population of large sensory fibers present at the points of stimulation. The fastest afferent cord potentials following posterior tibial nerve stimulation in the popliteal fossa (80 m/sec approximately) are largely absent when the same nerve is stimulated at the level of the ankle[3]. From this it can be concluded that the fast activity is likely to be due to afference of Groups I a and I b which derive from muscle spindles and tendon organs and are therefore present in much greater number at the level of the knee. Cutaneous fibers, mainly deriving from the distal extremities and therefore present in large number at the ankle also, seem to conduct rather more slowly in the cord (45–55 m/sec approximately).

S. J. JONES:

Refractory Period of Spinal SEP

Afferent spinal cord potentials remain virtually unaltered when the frequency of electrical stimulation is increased from 2 Hz to 20 Hz[3]. A fast stimulation rate naturally reduces the time taken acquiring an average and therefore helps provide the surgeon with rapid feedback. The effect of increasing the stimulation rate further has not been investigated, but an alternative method of determining the refractory period of spinal SEP is to stimulate at a regular, moderate frequency using a doublet impulse in which the interstimulus interval (ISI) can be systematically varied.

With ISIs of 10 msec or more the response to the second stimulus of the doublet is virtually identical to a single stimulus response, but at shorter intervals the investigation is hampered by the fact that earlier components in the response to the second stimulus begin to overlap with later potentials evoked by the first. It is therefore necessary to adopt a waveform subtraction technique and eliminate the response to the first stimulus by subtracting from the doublet waveform the potentials evoked by a single stimulus presented with the same frequency and intensity (Fig. 2).

With interstimulus intervals of less than 1 msec the entire response is virtually abolished, but between 1 and 4 msec there may be a differential effect on the 3 components with most marked attenuation of the first, fastest conducted potential (Fig. 2). This is not an intuitive finding, since

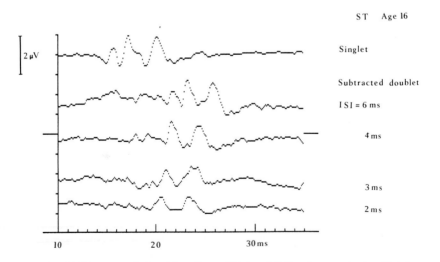

Fig. 2. Spinal SEPs recorded epidurally at T 1 level following posterior tibial nerve stimulation at the knee. Single stimuli were presented at 20/sec, plus doublets with ISI of 2–6 msec. Subtraction of the singlet waveform from each of the doublet responses shows the SEPs following the second stimulus of each doublet. Three components are identifiable in the latter at ISI = 6 msec, but the first is absent at ISI = 4, 3 and 2 msec

it is likely to be postsynaptic neurons which are more refractory at short ISI and one might have assumed that the activity of postsynaptic cord fibers (the relevant synapses being located in the dorsal horn at lumbosacral level) would have a *longer* latency at higher levels than that of fibers which are continued centrally without an intervening synapse. The finding, however, does tend to support the hypothesis that the initial, fastest conducted cord potentials are likely to be due to activation of Group I muscle and tendon afferents. Many of these are conducted centrally in the spinocerebellar tracts after synapsing in the dorsal horn, whereas a large proportion of Group II cutaneous fibers are continued in the dorsal columns without any synapse intervening.

Intensity of Stimulation

By slowly increasing the voltage of the applied stimulus, it can be demonstrated the 3 major components of the spinal SEP have different peripheral activation thresholds[3]. Axons of larger diameter and higher conduction velocity also have lower electrical thresholds, and this is consistent with the observation that the 3 components appear in order of increasing latency as the stimulus voltage is increased. This phenomenon may be used to distinguish the components from one another in the thoracic region where they overlap to a greater extent, and indeed may not occur in the same temporal sequence as at higher levels.

Pharmacologic Factors

For most practical purposes, anesthetic agents administered systemically in surgical concentrations may be assumed to have little effect on spinal SEPs, in contrast to the marked and varied effect of many agents on cortical evoked responses. This is not to say, however, that there may not be a small influence at spinal level (see, for example, 6) and this is likely to be greatest for postsynaptic neurons. It may be the case that anesthetics administered epidurally would have a more marked effect, although so far this appears not to have been investigated.

Effect of Temperature

When the vertebral column is exposed for long periods during surgery, a progressive increase in the latency of spinal SEPs is observed. At the upper thoracic level this seldom exceeds 1 msec, is seen to be rapidly reversible if the recording electrodes are left in place during closure, and appears to have no pathological consequences.

Pathologic Factors

Hypotension

In the great majority of operations, changes in blood pressure occurring either spontaneously or induced by pharmacologic manipulation have little effect on the amplitude or latency of spinal SEPs, in contrast to the marked attenuation of cortical evoked responses which occurs below approximately 80 mmHg. Profound hypotension below 40 mm Hg does result in conduction block due to ischemia of the cord[9], but if not unduly protracted appears to be fully reversible after restoration of normal blood pressure. Segmental potentials may be transiently enhanced in the ischemic cord[6], which may account for the observation by Whittle *et al.*[9] that a volume-conducted potential presumed to arise in the cord at the level of entry appeared or was increased in amplitude at the same time as conduction deficits were manifested more rostrally.

Cord Concussion

Minor concussion of the cord at the root entry level (the conus medullaris for lower limb responses) may cause transient attenuation or abolishment of spinal SEPs recorded more rostrally, and it appears that it may be postsynaptic potentials which are most susceptible (for example see Case 3, Fig. 3, of Jones *et al.*[4]). A possible mechanism might be one of synaptic depression caused by the release of potassium ions in the extracellular space and possibly similar to processes occurring during "spinal shock." The latter would seem to be a phenomenon worth investigating by spinal SEPs but so far has received little attention from electrophysiologists.

Distraction of the Spine

The deterioration of spinal SEPs caused by distraction of the vertebral column during scoliosis correction and the consequent neurological deficits if the impairment is not reversed are believed to be due to local ischemia rather than direct traction on the cord. The effect may not be manifested for some time after the event presumed to be responsible, and it is usually fully or partially reversible for at least 20 min after detection. In spinal SEP recordings there is no sure way of distinguishing the effect of impaired cord conduction from attenuation of the response due to movement of the electrode tip or diminution of stimulus intensity, and for this reason a decrement of up to 60% may have to be regarded as of doubtful significance. Increase in latency is seldom, if ever, an indication of impending conduction failure. However, the finding that spinal SEPs are more often reduced than increased in amplitude after distraction[4] suggests that a genuine, if sub-

clinical, conduction impairment may be produced in a substantial proportion of cases. It follows that the incidence of "false positives" may
actually be much lower than the proportion of cases in which apparent
deterioration of the SEP is not associated with any postoperative neurological deficit.

SEP deterioration following spinal distraction may be unilateral or
bilateral, so alternate stimulation of both legs is recommended. It may also
be useful to monitor activity below the level of the correction either pe-
riodically, or continuously if a second recording channel is available, to
exclude the possibility that a deteriorating response recorded more rostrally
is due to diminishing stimulus intensity or other technical factors. Although
the possibility exists that a defect confined to anterior spinal cord tracts
might be missed when only sensory potentials are monitored, there have
been no convincing reports of such cases in which spinal SEPs were recorded. Nevertheless, some form of efferent monitor is obviously desirable.
The most promising technique would seem to be that of recording the
descending volley following stimulation of the motor cortex through the
scalp[1].

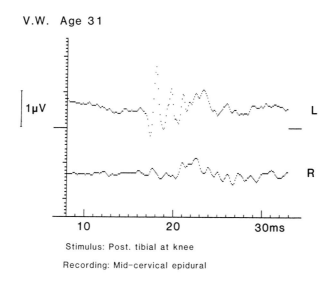

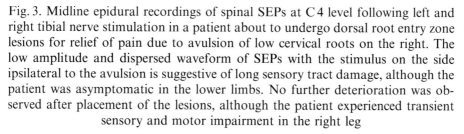

Fig. 3. Midline epidural recordings of spinal SEPs at C 4 level following left and
right tibial nerve stimulation in a patient about to undergo dorsal root entry zone
lesions for relief of pain due to avulsion of low cervical roots on the right. The
low amplitude and dispersed waveform of SEPs with the stimulus on the side
ipsilateral to the avulsion is suggestive of long sensory tract damage, although the
patient was asymptomatic in the lower limbs. No further deterioration was observed after placement of the lesions, although the patient experienced transient
sensory and motor impairment in the right leg

Pre-existing Neurological Lesions

The successful recording of spinal SEPs is greatly dependent on the coherence of the afferent volley. The response to tibial nerve stimulation recorded epi- or intradurally above C 5 level in patients who had suffered avulsion of lower cervical roots was frequently found to be of low amplitude and dispersed waveform on the ipsilateral side, although the patients were neurologically asymptomatic in the lower limbs[2]. In contrast to cortical SEPs, which can be detectable in the presence of severe peripheral neuropathy or spinal cord pathology, spinal SEPs may be very difficult to record where there is only mild pre-existing neurological impairment and so may be unsuited for monitoring such neurosurgical procedures as the excision of spinal tumors. Evoked spinal cord potentials are of much larger amplitude when the stimulus is delivered directly to the cord or cauda equina from the epidural space and may therefore be more easily monitored in the presence of a cord lesion[8].

Surgical Lesions

The placement of surgical lesions in the dorsal root entry zone of the spinal cord for the relief of pain due, for example, to root avulsions also frequently causes mild to moderate long tract impairment. It is surprising, therefore,

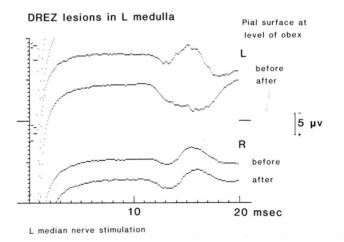

Fig. 4. Potentials recorded from the pial surface of the left and right medulla following left median nerve stimulation in a patient receiving dorsal root entry zone lesions on the left for relief of intractable pain due to trigeminal neuralgia. The potentials were initially more symmetrically recorded than in the patient illustrated in Fig. 1. The marked change in waveform on the ipsilateral side, consistent with a "killed end" or "injury" potential, was associated with weakness, ataxia and sensory loss

that continuous monitoring of spinal SEPs usually failed to demonstrate any significant defect immediately after the lesions were made[2] (Fig. 3). Most patients exhibited transient motor and sensory defects in the lower limbs postoperatively, and cortical SEPs recorded approximately 1 week later were usually significantly degraded in comparison with preoperative recordings. From this it was concluded that the impairment may have been a secondary (ischemic or inflammatory) consequence of surgical invasion of the cord. One patient in whom the lesions were made at the medullary level for intractable trigeminal pain showed a marked and immediate abnormality in pial-surface recordings (following median nerve stimulation) when the electrode was located on the ipsilateral side just above the level of the lesions, but not in more medial or contralateral recordings (Fig. 4). The substitution of a broad positive potential for the negativity recorded previously suggests a "killed-end" effect (sometimes termed an "injury potential"[7]) and it is possible that such changes might have been missed in earlier cases in which potentials were only recorded from the midline of the cord.

Acknowledgement

The work was performed in collaboration with Mr M. A. Edgar and Mr A. O. Ransford, Consultant Orthopaedic Surgeons at the Royal National Orthopaedic Hospital, and Mr D. G. T. Thomas, Consultant Neurosurgeon at the Hospital for Nervous Diseases.

References

1. Boyd SG, Cowan JMA, Rothwell JC, Webb PJ, Marsden CD (1985) Monitoring spinal motor tract function using cortical stimulation: a preliminary report. In: Schramm J, Jones SJ (eds) Spinal cord monitoring. Springer, Berlin Heidelberg New York Tokyo, pp 227–230
2. Jones SJ, Thomas DGT (1985) Assessment of long sensory tract conduction in patients undergoing dorsal root entry zone coagulation for pain relief. In: Schramm J, Jones SJ (eds) Spinal cord monitoring. Springer, Berlin Heidelberg New York Tokyo, pp 266–273
3. Jones SJ, Edgar MA, Ransford AO (1982) Sensory nerve conduction in the human spinal cord: epidural recordings made during scoliosis surgery. J Neurol Neurosurg Psychiatry 45: 446–451
4. Macon JB, Poletti CE (1982) Conducted somatosensory evoked potentials during spinal surgery. Part 1: Control conduction velocity measurements. J Neurosurg 57: 349–353
5. Shimoji K, Maruyama Y, Shimizu H, Fujioka H, Taga K (1985) Spinal cord monitoring – a review of current techniques and knowledge. In: Schramm J, Jones SJ (eds) Spinal cord monitoring. Springer, Berlin Heidelberg New York Tokyo, pp 16–28

6. Schramm J, Krause R, Shigeno T, Brock M (1984) Relevance of spinal cord evoked injury potential for spinal cord monitoring. In: Homma S, Tamaki T (eds) Fundamentals and clinical application of spinal cord monitoring. Saikon Publishing Co, Tokyo, pp 113–124
7. Takano H, Tamaki T, Noguchi T, Takakuwa K (1985) Comparison of spinal cord potentials elicited by spinal cord and peripheral nerve stimulation. In: Schramm J, Jones SJ (eds) Spinal cord monitoring. Springer, Berlin Heidelberg New York Tokyo, pp 29–34
8. Whittle IR, Johnson IH, Besser M (1986) Recording of spinal somatosensory evoked potentials for intraoperative spinal cord monitoring. J Neurosurg 64: 601–612

Somatosensory Evoked Potential Monitoring During Cervical Spine Surgery

A. Landi, A. Ducati, M. Cenzato, E. Fava*, D. Arvanitakis, D. Mulazzi**

Institute of Neurosurgery and * CNR Institute of Muscle Physiology, c/o Institute of Neurosurgery, ** II Chair of Anesthesiology, University of Milano (Italy)

Introduction

Cervical spine surgery poses risks of damage to the spinal cord and nerve roots[5]. Furthermore, either the arterial blood supply (anterior spinal artery and posterior radicular arteries) or the venous drainage (peridural plexus) may be damaged or stretched during surgical manipulation, producing an ischemic spinal cord injury. Therefore, it seems of interest to monitor spinal cord or nerve root function intraoperatively. Evoked potentials can detect spinal cord damage due to compression or ischemia[1]. Several authors have used somatosensory evoked potentials (SEPs) for monitoring during spinal surgery[2, 3, 4, 6, 7].

We report the use of intraoperative SEP monitoring during neurosurgical procedures on the cervical spine, including decompressive laminectomies, tumor ablations, and anterior discectomies and corpectomies.

The SEP data are correlated with surgical and anesthetic manoeuvres and with neurological outcome.

Materials and Methods

We studied 27 patients undergoing cervical spine surgery (2 intramedullary tumors, 4 extramedullary tumors, 10 decompressive laminectomies, 11 discectomies/corpectomies). Sixteen patients were males and 11 were females. Their average age was 40 years.

Anesthesia was induced with sodium thiopental 5–7 mg/kg and succinylcholine 1 mg/kg, then maintained with nitrous oxide 60% in oxygen and enflurane 0.8 to 1%. Under these conditions, it was always possible to record useful SEPs throughout the surgical procedures. The electrocardiogram (ECG), arterial pressure and heart rate were monitored continuously. Arterial pO_2, pCO_2, pH and plasma electrolytes were measured at intervals. Esophageal temperature was maintained between 35.8 and 36.3 °C. Surgery via an anterior approach was conducted on supine patients, while for the posterior approach patients were in the sitting position with the head flexed on the neck.

SEPs were recorded by means of commercial devices (Amplaid MK 10 and Amplaid MK 15). Using subdermal stainless steel needle electrodes, electrical stimuli were applied bilaterally to the posterior tibial nerves at ankles to obtain maximal fiber recruitment along spinal tracts and in cortical sensory areas. The median and ulnar nerves were stimulated at the wrist. Stimulus intensity was about 20 mA. In all cases, this level exceeded 3 times the threshold for a motor response, as measured in each patient before the use of muscle relaxants. Square wave impulses were delivered at one pulse per second (pps) and four pps for cortical and short latency SEPs (CSEPs and SSEPs), respectively. Pulse duration was 0.2 msec. Recordings were obtained using subdermal platinum needle electrodes. Recording channels for lower limb stimulation were as follows: L 2 ($+$) to iliac crest ($-$) and CZ to FpZ ($-$), with a ground electrode at the thigh. For upper limbs, recordings were from Erb's point ($+$) to FpZ ($-$) and C 3' or C 4' ($+$) to FpZ ($-$), with a ground electrode at the arm. Recording electrode impedances were 5 KOhm or less. Interelectrode impedances were maintained below 2 KOhm.

Traces were acquired with automatic artifact rejection. For lower limbs 1,000 responses were averaged on a 60 msec time base with a filter bandwidth of 10 to 2,500 Hz for short latency spinal and cortical recordings, and on a 200 msec time base with a filter bandwidth of 1 to 200 Hz for cortical recordings.

For upper limbs, 500 responses were averaged on a 30 msec time base with a filter bandwidth of 10 to 2,500 Hz for short latency Erb's point or cortical recordings and on a 200 msec time base with a filter bandwidth of 1 to 200 Hz for cortical recordings.

We measured the interpeak latency between lumbar or Erb's point waves and cortical waves. For stimulation at the ankle we calculated the spinal cord conduction velocity. For stimulation at the wrist, we determined the brachial plexus to cortex conduction time. In addition, we examined the amplitude and morphology of cortical waves.

Reference traces were obtained in each anesthetized patient before surgery. During surgery, SEPs were recorded every ten minutes. Continual recordings were performed during the critical phases. Each trace was plotted with related surgical and anesthetic data.

Data were analyzed by comparing SEP results with anesthetic, physiologic and surgical events during the operative procedure and with postoperative neurological outcome.

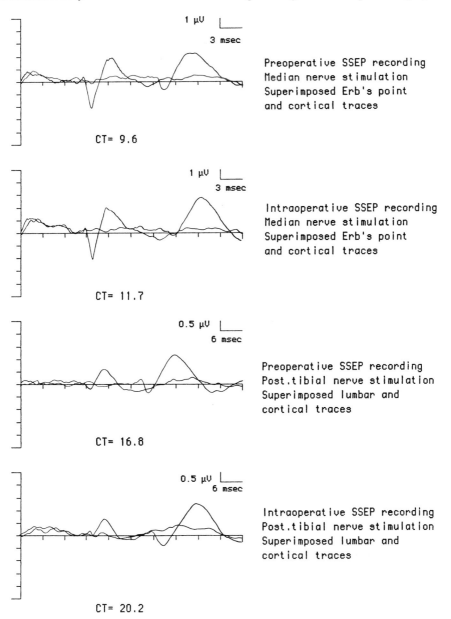

Fig. 1. Patient G. R., undergoing posterior decompressive laminectomy for cervical myelopathy due to spondylosis. Good improvement after surgery (Feb. 7, 1986). Stimulation of median nerve and of posterior tibial nerve alternatively. Recording sites are Erb's point and C 3′ or C 4′ referred to FpZ for median nerve stimulation; L 1/iliac crest and CZ/FpZ for posterior tibial nerve stimulation. Negativity downward

Results

The clinical features of the patients before surgery were as follows: 25 presented with paraparesis or lower limb monoparesis, sphincter dysfunction and sensory impairments such as paresthesia, hypesthesia and anesthesia. Five of these were quadriparetic. Two patients had no neurological deficits and were operated upon to stabilize the spine.

Postoperative outcome was good in 12 patients (44.4%), fair in 6 patients (22.2%), and unchanged in 7 patients (25.9%). Two patients (7.4%) suffered further neurological deterioration.

SSEPs and CSEPs showed different patterns of change intraoperatively. Lumbar and Erb's point responses were scarcely affected by anesthetic agents and changes in arterial blood pressure. In all our cases these waveforms were recorded without modification during the whole intervention; their latencies were compatible with normal peripheral nerve conduction velocities.

During surgery, distraction and compression upon the spine or its vessels increased the latency of the cortical wave (up to 12 msec from lower limbs and 6 msec from upper limbs) and decreased amplitude down to the disappearance of the response. Loss of the response was reversible in all cases but one within 10 minutes, provided that distraction was removed.

A suggestive correlation between the clinical outcome and the rank of intraoperative SSEP changes was found.

Among the 18 clinically improved patients we observed, during the critical decompression phases of surgery, a latency increase in the cortical waves not longer than 7 msec from lower limb stimulation and not longer than 3 msec from upper limb stimulation. These changes never lasted longer than 5 minutes (Fig. 1).

Amplitudes were more readily evaluated by recording the entire cortical response, than with the short-latency response alone. In no case did we see a reduction in amplitude more than 25% of the reference trace. After cord and root decompression in 11 cases the response was larger and had a shorter latency than in the beginning. A response was judged larger if, under the same conditions of body temperature and anesthetic concentration, its amplitude exceeded that of the reference trace by at least 20%. In the remaining 7 patients the response was unchanged.

Among the seven patients with no change in neurological function after surgery, conduction time during decompression never increased more than 3 msec from upper limb stimulation or more than 7 msec from lower limb stimulation. Thus, these patients showed the same increase in conduction time as the preceding group. On the other hand, the amplitude of the cortical response in these patients always decreased 30 to 50% during decompression and never showed any significant improvement, as compared to reference traces, after decompression.

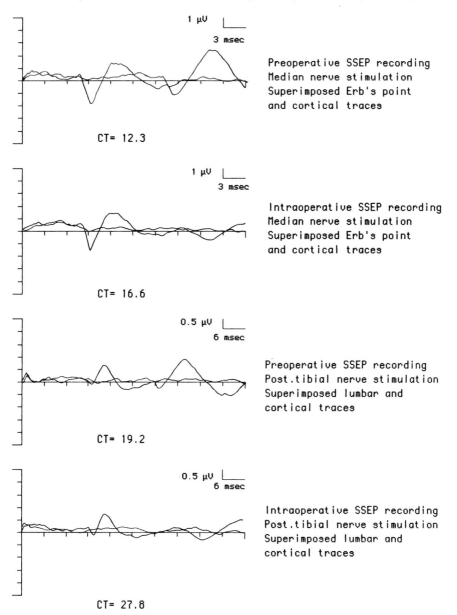

Fig. 2. Patient C. N., operated upon for an intramedullar astrocytoma. Severe deterioration after surgery (Nov. 7, 1985). Stimulation, recording sites and polarity as in Fig. 1

The two patients with postoperative deterioration had intraoperative prolongations of the conduction time of more than 3 and 7 msec for upper and lower limb stimulation, respectively, to 6 and 12 msec. The amplitude at the end of surgery was lost in one patient and severely decreased in the other (Fig. 2).

Discussion

According to other authors' reports[3, 7], SEP recording seems to be a reliable method for intraoperative monitoring during cervical spine surgery.

In our series a prolongation of the conduction time of no more than 3 and 7 msec from upper and lower limb stimulation, respectively, is a good indicator that the patient will not show postoperative deterioration. The amplitude of the responses, recorded after decompression of the cord or the nerve roots, seems to be the most reliable indicator of possible clinical improvement. However, good clinical outcomes were also seen in patients who did not show an amplitude increase after bony decompression; in these cases, the maximal amplitude reduction during decompression was 25% of baseline.

On the other hand, patients with prolongations of conduction time more than 7 msec and 3 msec, respectively, for lower and upper limb stimulation, invariably showed postoperative deterioration especially if cortical responses disappeared intraoperatively. No falsely pessimistic results were seen.

In agreement with other authors[3, 4], we conclude that both latency increases and amplitude decreases of cortical waves are significant in the evaluation of the neural damage occurring during surgery. The prudent limits we report are wider than others in the literature[4]. The wider range of SEP changes we noted may have been due to local cooling of the cord, caused by long exposure and frequent saline irrigation.

We made several observations relating to specific surgical problems.

Removal of intramedullary tumors requires posterior column splitting and dissection. Since SEPs are mainly conducted along lemniscal pathways, they might disappear due to a traumatic blockage of conduction. We believe that disappearance of the cortical responses suggests that the acute cord damage has been so severe that a neurological deterioration can be expected postoperatively. Possibly, recordings carried out using electrodes placed directly over the spinal cord might provide a more direct demonstration of the cord damage.

SEPs are predominantly conducted through the dorsal columns in the posterior quadrants of the spinal cord[9]. It would be of interest to evaluate the activity of the sensory pathways running in the anterior quadrants of the spinal cord, close to the descending motor pathways. The anterior sensory pathways are possibly activated only with a very high stimulus intensity. We never reached the stimulus intensity needed to activate these fibers, reported in an experimental work to be 30 times the motor threshold[8].

Finally, we think that the amplitude increase resulting from bone removal might be more properly attributed to root decompression than to decompression of the cord.

References

1. Bennet M (1983) Effect of compression and ischemia on spinal cord evoked potentials. Exp Neurol 80: 508–519
2. Grundy BL (1982) Monitoring of Sensory Evoked Potentials during neurosurgical operations: Methods and applications. Neurosurg 11-4: 556–576
3. Grundy BL, Nelson PB, Doyle E, Procopio PT (1982) Intraoperative loss of somatosensory evoked potentials predicts loss of spinal cord function. Anesthesiology 57: 321–322
4. Hahn JGF, Latchaw JP (1983) Evoked potentials in the operating room. Clin Neurosurg 31: 389–403
5. Hoff JT (1985) Cervical disc disease and cervical spondylosis. In: Wilkins RH, Rengachary SS (eds) Neurosurgery. McGraw Hill Book Co, New York, pp 2230–2239
6. Macon JB, Poletti CE (1982) Conducted somatosensory evoked potentials during spinal surgery. Part 1: Control conduction velocity measurements. J Neurosurg 57: 349–353
7. Macon JB, Poletti CE, Ojemann WH, Zervas NT (1982) Conducted somatosensory evoked potentials during spinal surgery. Part 2: Clinical applications. J Neurosurg 57: 354–359
8. Schieppati M, Ducati A (1981) Effects of stimulus intensity, cervical cord tractotomies and cerebellectomy on Somatosensory evoked potentials from skin and muscle afferents of cat hind limbs. Electroencephalogr Clin Neurophysiol 51: 363–372
9. Simpson RK, Jr, Blackburn JB, Martin HF, Katz S (1981) Peripheral nerve fiber and spinal cord pathways contributions to the Somatosensory evoked potentials. Exp Neurol 73: 700–715

BAEP and SSEP Monitoring During Posterior Fossa Surgery

A. Ducati, A. Landi, M. Cenzato, E. Fava*, A. Parma**,
M. Giovanelli

Institute of Neurosurgery and * CNR Institute of Muscle Physiology, c/o Institute of Neurosurgery, ** II Chair of Anesthesiology, University of Milano (Italy)

Introduction

Posterior fossa surgery carries two different classes of risks:
— those connected with the sitting position (when this position is used);
— those connected with the approach to tumors or vascular malformations of this region, where many vital neural structures are contained in a very limited space.

These risks have been so difficult to cope with that, in the early years of neurological surgery, the mortality rate was intolerably high. Harvey Cushing in the 1930s described the cerebellopontine angle, where most of the surgically treatable tumors are seated, as the "gloomy corner of neurological surgery." The need for a monitoring system is therefore particularly high in posterior fossa surgery.

Evoked potential (EP) monitoring has recently been introduced as part of the clinical routine. Evoked responses may change intraoperatively as a consequence of anesthesiological or surgical procedures.

The anesthesiologist uses other monitoring systems to help control many physiological parameters, but still some problems remain. For instance, an arterial blood pressure value that is normally sufficient to maintain a good cerebral perfusion may not be adequate to provide suitable cerebral circulation in a specific patient. The surgeon has no way to directly evaluate the clinical neurological function of patients under general anesthesia.

Evoked potential monitoring permits, at least, the evaluation of conduction through specific acoustic and somatosensory pathways in an unconscious patient. Indirect information is available concerning the nervous system structure that contains the sensory pathways, in this case the brainstem.

To make EP monitoring satisfactory for enhancing patient safety during posterior fossa surgery, some basic points must be considered:

a) The reliability of the technique in identifying functional lesions of the brainstem or of other nervous system structures must be determined in terms of falsely optimistic and falsely pessimistic results.

b) The sensitivity of the technique must be sufficient to detect lesions while they are still reversible, provided suitable measures are taken.

c) The tolerance limits of a conduction change required to correctly predict the postoperative outcome, either favorable or unfavorable, must be determined.

Methods and Material

41 of the 72 patients who underwent posterior fossa surgery at our institution during the last 3 years were monitored by using evoked potentials: 25 patients had neurinomas of cranial nerve VIII; 5 patients had meningiomas of the posterior wall of the petrous bone; 7 had cerebellar tumors (astrocytomas and medulloblastomas); and 4 had vascular malformations.

Evoked potentials were recorded by means of commercial systems (Amplaid MK 10 and Amplaid MK 15).

8 patients were studied using acoustic stimulation only; 33 had both brainstem auditory EP (BAEP) and short-latency somatosensory EP (SSEP) recording. The reason for this change in the recording protocol was that in our series several large neurinomas (diameter > 3 cm) were present, so that, in the preoperative recording, not only was the response ipsilateral to the tumor absent, but, even upon contralateral stimulation, no evoked activity could be consistently recorded.

Besides, as suggested by Little et al.[5], the bimodality approach achieves better evaluation of brainstem function.

Acoustic stimulation was carried out using the ordinary headphones, with an intensity 20 dB more than that used for preoperative recording.

The recording electrodes – platinum subdermal needles – were placed on the vertex and on the earlobes. The time of analysis was 12 msec, with a filter bandwidth of 100–2,500 Hz, and a stimulation frequency of 11 pulses per second. Higher frequencies gave inconsistent results during anesthesia.

The I to V interpeak latency (IPL) (normal accepted values less than 4.5 msec) and the amplitude ratio between wave V and wave I (normally > 1) were measured.

Somatosensory stimulation was achieved by bilateral median nerve electrical shocks at an intensity of 20 mA, delivered by subdermal stainless steel needle electrodes. This value exceeded three times threshold for motor twitch (measured before the use of muscle relaxants). The recording electrodes – platinum subdermal needles – were placed over Erb's point and on the scalp overlying the sensory cortex (C 3' or C 4', just posterior to the C 3 and C 4 positions of the international 10–20 EEG system[4]). Both channels were referred to FpZ. A cervical electrode was never employed, because it was so close to the surgical field that it was not possible to guarantee a reasonable recording. SSEPs were recorded on a 30 msec time base, with a filter bandwidth of 10–2,500 Hz and a stimulus frequency of 4 pulses per second. The somatosensory conduction time (CT) was calculated as the difference between N 20 latency and Erb's point latency. The maximum accepted value of somatosensory CT was 11 msec, with a maximum interhemispheric difference of 0.6 msec.

Preoperative recordings were obtained the day before surgery. A reference trace for both BAEPs and SSEPs was obtained when the patient was in the final surgical position and in a well established and constant level of anesthesia.

Esophageal temperature was recorded, and measured values ranged form 35.5 to 36 °C.

The patients were premedicated with hydroxyzine hydrochloride 200 mg and atropine 0.5 mg, given intramuscularly. Anesthesia was induced with sodium thiopental 3–5 mg/kg and succinylcholine 0.1 mg/kg facilitated endotracheal intubation. Ventilation was controlled with a Siemens SERVO-VENTILATOR 900 C to maintain $paCO_2$ at 30 mmHg throughout the surgical procedure. Anesthesia was maintained with oxygen in 60% nitrous oxide, enflurane 1.4% end-expired, and intravenous fentanyl, 0.05 mg, as needed.

Results

In the preoperative recordings, 12 patients presented with normal responses to both acoustic and somatosensory stimulation. This group included all cases with cerebellar tumors and vascular malformations of the vertebral-basilar system.

The other 29 patients, with neurinomas or meningiomas of the ponto-cerebellar angle, all had abnormal BAEPs; moreover, 20 of the 21 examined subjects also had a prolonged somatosensory CT, either in terms of absolute value (*i.e.*, longer than 11 msec) or in terms of interhemispheric difference (*i.e.*, greater than 0.6 msec).

One of the 12 patients presenting with cerebellar tumors and with vascular malformations of the vertebral-basilar system, on the first recording during anesthesia in the sitting position, showed a prolongation of the somatosensory CT exceeding 2 msec as compared to the preoperative recordings. This prolongation of conduction time exceeds what is normally seen as a consequence of anesthetic agents and hypothermia. The patient's mean arterial blood pressure was 90 mmHg, and this was judged possibly insufficient to satisfactorily perfuse the hemispheres. The patient was returned to the supine position and the response recovered in 15 minutes. Surgery went on uneventfully with arterial blood pressure maintained at

BAEP recording upon stimulation of the left ear and ipsilateral recording

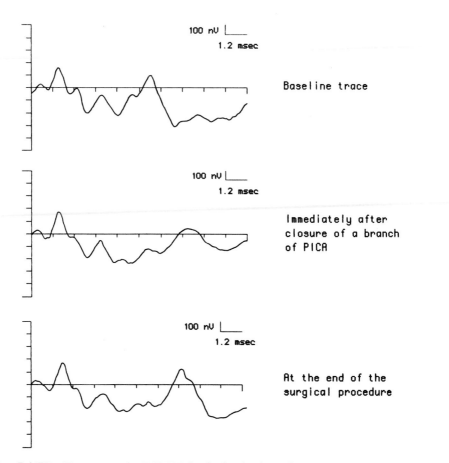

Fig. 1 a. BAEPs. Top trace: the I-V IPL in the beginning of surgery is at the upper limit of normal (4.5 msec). Middle trace: after closure of a branch of the posterior inferior cerebellar artery (PICA), a sudden increase of the I-V IPL takes place, to 6.8 msec. Bottom trace: The change persists until the end of the surgical procedure

a higher level. BAEPs were subsequently unchanged throughout recording in this patient.

No significant change took place at the beginning of surgery in the 11 other patients with normal preoperative recordings. In 6, when the dura mater of the posterior fossa was opened and CSF removed from the cisterns, a small but persistent shortening of the I-V interpeak latency and of SSEP CT was noted. In one patient, a sudden intraoperative increase in latency

SSEPs upon right median nerve stimulation: recording from
right Erb's point and from C3' (versus Fp2)

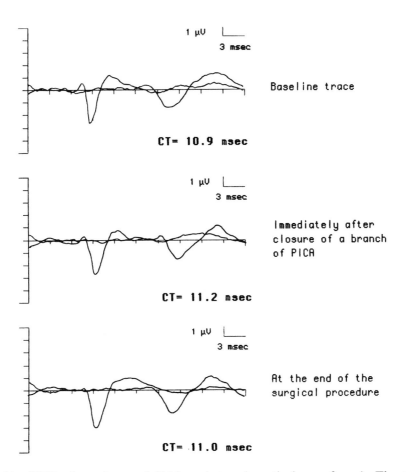

Fig. 1 b. SSEPs (superimposed Erb's point and cortical waveforms). The top, middle and bottom traces were recorded immediately after the corresponding BAEP traces of (a). No significant change in the somatosensory CT is evident. Negativity downward

and a slight reduction in amplitude of BAEP wave V took place on the side where a branch of the PICA was occluded during tumor dissection. This modification did not recover during surgery. The somatosensory CT remained unchanged (Fig. 1 a and b). The patient awoke without any new neurological deficit and was discharged after an uneventful postoperative course. The other patients in this group did not show any significant intraoperative worsening of evoked responses, and their postoperative courses were uneventful.

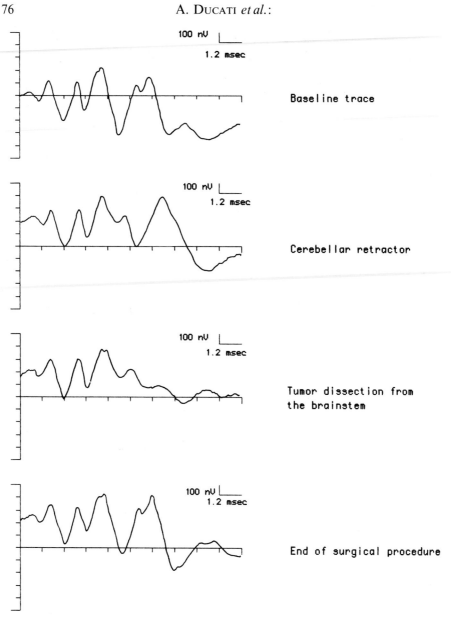

Fig. 2. BAEPs. Top: the I-V IPL at the beginning of surgery is prolonged. Second: the placement of a cerebellar retractor causes a further increase of the I-V IPL. Third: tumor dissection from the brainstem makes wave V hardly recognizable. Interruption of surgical manipulation allows the trace to recover. Bottom: at the end of the procedure the BAEP response is comparable to that obtained in the beginning

As stated above, the 29 patients affected by neurinomas or by meningiomas of the cerebellopontine angle presented with abnormal preoperative EPs.

The limitation of intraoperative BAEP recording during resection of posterior fossa neurinomas is that most patients have severe hearing loss (all those with neurinomas in our series and 2 with meningiomas). A reliable trace upon stimulation on the side of the tumor was never achievable during surgery. Moreover, even the contralateral trace, upon stimulation of the sound ear, was hardly obtainable during surgery. Therefore, all our traces refer to the ipsilateral recording when stimulating the sound ear: they are contralateral to the tumor side and may be considered as a monitor of the brainstem itself, not of the acoustic nerve.

These recordings proved to be useful in identifying the most critical events during surgery. In 15 patients, placement of a cerebellar retractor caused a slight but persistent prolongation of the I-V IPL (Fig. 2 top and second trace), in 2 cases as great as 1.5 msec. This change was reversible when the retractor was removed. It is difficult to understand the pathophysiology of this alteration: its abrupt onset suggests that a mechanical distortion is more likely than a vascular (possibly venous) impairment.

The dissection of the median wall of the tumor from the brainstem caused, in most cases, a change of the morphology and latency of the response, particularly of wave V (Fig. 2, third trace). In 3 cases, wave V was hardly visible for 10 minutes. The change of wave V always appeared before the clinical signs of brainstem impairment, such as bradycardia or heart rate alterations. Wave V recovered its latency, amplitude and morphology within the time of the surgery, and the patients awakened normally.

In another patient, the BAEP trace showed a progressive change during tumor dissection that ended in complete loss of the response except for wave I. The patient showed no other sign of brainstem failure, and surgery proceeded. However, the patient never awoke and he died 15 days after surgery. Unfortunately, this was one of the first patients undergoing intraoperative EP monitoring, and we did not record the somatosensory response.

When the BAEP is used to monitor brainstem function and not just the acoustic nerve, a normal waveform at the end of surgery is a reliable sign that the patient will survive. On the other hand, if the BAEP trace is lost, the patient will most likely present with postoperative disorders of consciousness.

The integrity of BAEPs, however, is not sufficient to predict a good postoperative course without further neurological deficits. One patient demonstrated this fact dramatically. During the course of the surgery, the acoustic response contralateral to the tumor side never showed any significant change, and at the end of the operation a response was even present

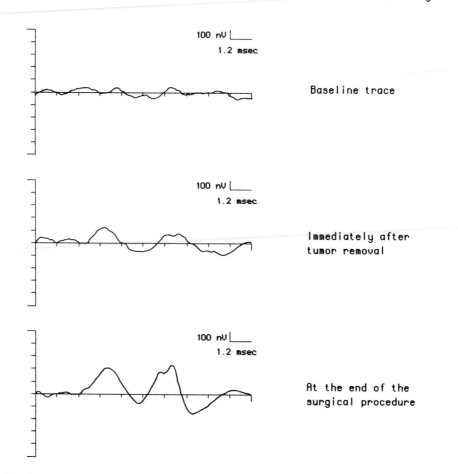

BAEPs upon stimulation of the left ear and contralateral recording

100 nV

1.2 msec

Baseline trace

100 nV

1.2 msec

Immediately after tumor removal

100 nV

1.2 msec

At the end of the surgical procedure

Fig. 3 a. BAEPs. Top: no response is recordable on the side of the tumor during stimulation of the contralateral ear at the beginning of surgery. Middle: after removal of the neurinoma, some consistent activity appears. Bottom: 30 minutes later, at the end of the surgical procedure, a morphologically normal trace, although still showing a marked latency increase

on the side of the tumor upon stimulation of the sound ear (Fig. 3 a). Somatosensory potentials, on the other hand, did show changes (Fig. 3 b). While in the beginning of surgery the interhemispheric difference of conduction time was 1.5 msec, the latency of the cortical response on the side of the tumor progressively increased and reached an interhemispheric difference of 4.2 msec. Moreover, the amplitude of the response decreased on the pathological side. Although noticed and discussed, this change in somatosensory conduction was not correctly evaluated, principally because

SSEPs upon left median nerve stimulation: recording from
Erb's point and from C4' (versus Fp2)

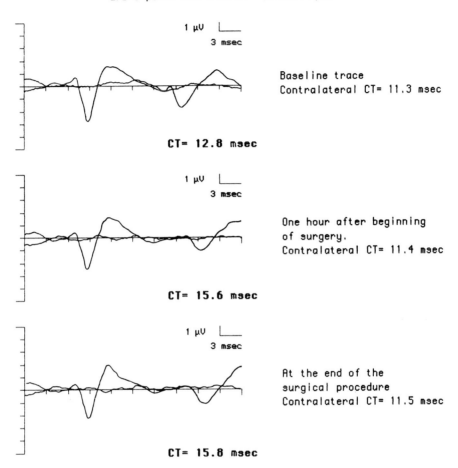

Baseline trace
Contralateral CT= 11.3 msec

CT= 12.8 msec

One hour after beginning
of surgery.
Contralateral CT= 11.4 msec

CT= 15.6 msec

At the end of the
surgical procedure
Contralateral CT= 11.5 msec

CT= 15.8 msec

Fig. 3 b. SSEPs (superimposed Erb's point and cortical responses). Top: in the beginning of surgery, the interhemispheric difference of somatosensory CT is 1.5 msec. Middle: one hour after, there is a significant increase of CT difference, to as long as 4.2 msec. Bottom: the CT difference persists to the end of surgery. The patient awakened with a dense hemiparesis. Negativity downward

of the normality of the BAEP traces. At the end of surgery, the patient presented with a dense, persisting hemiparesis contralateral to the affected hemisphere. The explanation of this dramatic conclusion was not fully understood; it is likely, however, that rotation of the head caused a critical reduction of blood flow in the extracranial carotid artery. In fact, the postoperative CT demonstrated a hypodensity in the white matter consistent with an ischemic infarction.

In conclusion, among this group of patients, one died in the postoperative course without ever regaining consciousness; he showed a loss of BAEPs during surgery. Another patient, with normal BAEPs and prolonged SSEP conduction time, suffered a severe and persisting motor disability. All the other subjects, with only minor and transient change of EP traces, recovered and had a normal postoperative course.

Discussion

The value of BAEP monitoring to preserve acoustic function during resection of very small acoustic neurinomas is well known[2]. Our results stress the importance of BAEP monitoring to evaluate brainstem function during resection of very large tumors of the cerebellopontine angle. Under these conditions, the disappearance of BAEP traces points to severe brainstem involvement, which, in our experience, has not been compatible with patient survival. Similar results have been reported by Raudzens[6]. On the other hand, no patient with normal traces during the whole surgical procedure, or with only minor and reversible changes, experienced postoperative disorders of consciousness. Moreover, in one case (cerebellar astrocytoma) a prolongation of the I to V interpeak latency of more than 2 msec, in presence of a normal and unchanged somatosensory conduction time was not followed by any clinical complication in the postoperative course.

As far as hemispheric function is concerned, BAEPs cannot obviously provide any useful information[3]. A dramatic prolongation of the somatosensory CT is compatible with an unchanged BAEP and points either to supratentorial dysfunction, as in our patient, or, possibly, to a cervicomedullary lesion. These two severe complications of posterior fossa surgery, carried out in the sitting position, are rare but well known and dreaded. They can usually be prevented by avoiding excessive rotation and flexion of the head[1]. For this purpose, the comparison between preoperative and intraoperative EP recording may be extremely helpful.

The EP changes observed intraoperatively were fully reversible when suitable corrective measures were taken within 2 or 3 minutes after the change had appeared. This fact can be interpreted as if the lesion documented by EPs is only functional, not yet structural, at least in the beginning. It is not known how long it takes to evolve into an anatomical, irreversible change. In 3 patients, however, we observed a loss or a severe reduction of wave V for 10 minutes, with neither persistent change of the EPs nor worsening of the clinical signs after surgery. For SSEPs, an interhemispheric difference of 2 msec was compatible with full postoperative recovery, while in the patient exhibiting an interhemispheric difference of 4.2 msec a dense and persisting hemiparesis ensued.

References

1. Buchheit WA, Delgado TE (1985) Tumors of the cerebellopontine angle: clinical features and surgical management. In: Wilkins and Rengachary (eds) Neurosurgery, Part VI: Neuro-oncology. Mc Graw-Hill Book Company, New York, pp 7–729
2. Grundy BL, Lina A, Procopio PT, Jannetta PJ (1982) Reversible evoked potential changes with retraction of the eighth cranial nerve. Anesth Analg (Cleveland) 61: 186–187
3. Grundy BL (1983) Intraoperative monitoring of sensory-evoked potentials. Anesthesiology 58: 72–87
4. Jasper HH (1958) The ten twenty electrode system of the International Federation. Electroencephalogr Clin Neurophysiol 10: 371–375
5. Little JR, Zesser RP, Lueders H, Furlan AJ (1983) Brainstem acoustic evoked potentials in posterior circulation surgery. Neurosurgery 12: 496–502
6. Raudzens PA (1982) Intraoperative monitoring of evoked potentials. Ann NY Acad Sci 388: 308–326

Intraoperative Monitoring of Sensory Evoked Potentials in Cerebellopontine Angle Tumors

L. Lutzemberger, G. Tusini

Institute of Neurosurgery, University of Pisa (Italy)

Monitoring of brainstem neurophysiological functions by the recording of objective parameters may be of considerable help during neurosurgical operations within the posterior fossa. Postoperative neurological deficits may be secondary to mechanical traction or to compression of nervous tissue; such damage may be avoided if functional deterioration is recognized and promptly corrected before irreversible structural alterations occur.

The brainstem auditory evoked potentials (BAEPs) reflect the sequential activation of several neural generators in the pons and in the mesencephalon; they are a useful means of exploring brainstem function[3, 7, 8]. Some characteristics make BAEPs particularly indicated for the intraoperative monitoring; the waves are stable and reproducible; they can be recorded by scalp electrodes without interfering with the surgical field; BAEP components are easily recorded under anesthesia and are resistant to the effects of most anesthetic agents. Therefore, this technique is often utilized in the operating room to monitor brainstem function during posterior fossa surgery[1, 2, 4, 6]. In this paper intraoperative BAEP alterations during the removal of 23 cerebellopontine angle tumors are described (Table 1).

A relevant point in functional monitoring of the brainstem by intraoperative BAEP recording is that a normal conduction of the acoustic signal cannot be extrapolated to prove the integrity of the entire brainstem.

In recent work, Piatt et al.[5] demonstrated in one patient the insensitivity of intraoperative BAEP monitoring to compromised brainstem function. In order to explore a larger area of the brainstem during posterior fossa surgery, function of the somatosensory pathways can be monitored by recording somatosensory evoked potentials (SEPs) in addition to BAEPs. Brainstem function is still only partially monitored, but the probability of revealing intraoperative alterations related to one system or to the other is certainly increased.

Methods

In 23 patients undergoing surgery for cerebellopontine angle tumors, BAEPs were monitored, intraoperatively. In 9 of these cases, SEPs were recorded at the same time (Table 1).

For BAEP recording, electrodes were placed on each mastoid and on the vertex, with a forehead electrode acting as ground. A vertex-positive wave was recorded as an upgoing wave. Clicks were generated by passing 0.1 msec square-wave pulses at a rate of 10/sec through headphones to produce alternating rarefaction and condensation sound pressure waves. Stimulation intensity was adjusted to 80 dB above the hearing threshold of the tested ear. High-pass and low-pass filters were set at 150 and 2,000 Hz, respectively. A time of 100 sec was generally sufficient to record a clear signal by the averaging of 1,000 repetitions.

Intraoperative monitoring of the brainstem was performed by recording BAEPs contralateral to the tumor. The large size of the cerebellopontine angle tumors had caused total loss of ipsilateral hearing in most cases. In the few cases in which hearing was preserved, distortion of BAEPs due to surgical manipulation of the 8th nerve hampered monitoring of the auditory nerve and brainstem.

SEPs were elicited by percutaneous electrical stimulation of the median nerve at the wrist. Square wave pulses of 0.3 msec duration and 5/sec frequency were used. Stimulus intensity was three times twitch threshold. Cortical and subcortical SEPs were recorded by electrodes placed 2 cm behind Cz and on the spinous process of the second cervical vertebra (CS 2), with reference at Fz of the International 10/20 system. Electrode impedance was maintained at less than 5,000 ohms. The recording bandwidth was 5 to 800 Hz; 256 responses were averaged. SEPs were recorded on an Interspec Neurotrac.

Table 1

Cerebellopontine angle operations monitored by evoked potentials	BAEP monitoring	SEP monitoring	BAEP alterations	SEP alterations
Acoustic neurinomas	15	5	2	–
Trigeminal neurinomas	2	1	1	–
Hypoglosseal neurinomas	1	1	–	1
Meningiomas	5	2	2	1
	23	9	5	2

Systemic blood pressure, arterial pH, pCO_2 and pO_2, plasma osmolality, and body temperature were recorded at frequent intervals.

Evoked potentials were recorded at intervals of 2–3 minutes and superimposed on one another for comparison. Alterations of evoked responses were immediately reported to the surgeon for possible modification of surgical dissection or adjustment of retractors.

Results

Intraoperative changes in evoked potentials were identified in 6 cases during tumor dissection or deep cerebellar retraction (Table 1). In all cases evoked potentials returned to baseline levels within 6 to 25 minutes after modification of dissection or readjustment of the retractor. After operation, no neurological signs of the brainstem impairment were present.

Intraoperative BAEP changes always referred to wave V, which in two cases showed a progressive latency increase of more than 1 msec with amplitude attenuation. In three cases, wave V was completely lost. For example, Fig. 1 shows loss of wave V during deep retraction followed by return of the wave 8 minutes after removal of the retractor.

Both BAEP and SEP deteriorated intraoperatively in one case (Fig. 2),

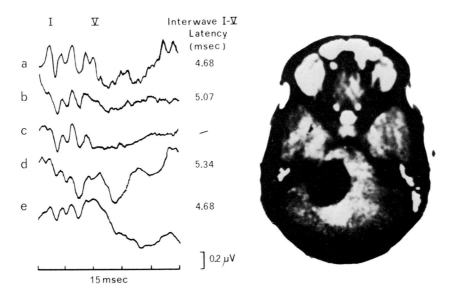

Fig. 1. Effects on BAEPs of deep cerebellar retraction during the removal of an acoustic neurinoma. (a) control; (b) and (c) recordings performed 2 and 3 minutes after retractor placement; (d) and (e) BAEP recordings 8 and 10 minutes after retractor removal

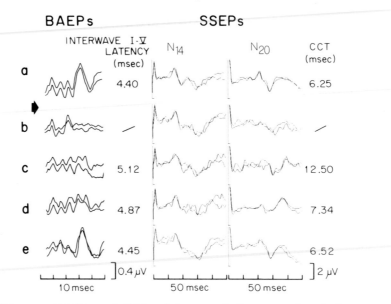

Fig. 2. Effects on BAEPs and SEPs of deep cerebellar retraction during removal of a meningioma. The arrow indicates the placement of the retractor. (a) control; (b) BAEPs and SEPs recorded after 3 minutes of deep retraction; (c, d), and (e) BAEP and SEP recordings 4, 10, and 18 minutes after retractor removal

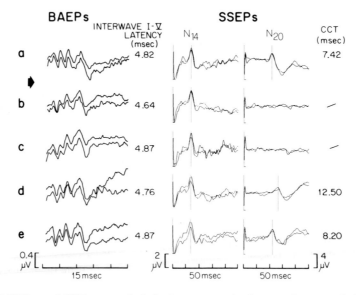

Fig. 3. BAEPs and SEPs recorded during removal of a neurinoma of the hypoglosseal nerve. (a) control; (b) 2 minutes after the beginning of tumor dissection from the brainstem, the SEP N 20 was completely lost. (c, d), and (e) BAEPs and SEPs recorded 2, 10, and 20 minutes after interruption of dissection. BAEP recordings showed no alteration

in association with brainstem compression. After retractor removal, evoked potentials recovered to normal over the next 18 minutes.

In another patient (Fig. 3), clear intraoperative dissociation between BAEP and SEP developed during dissection of a large neurinoma of the hypoglosseal nerve. While no BAEP changes appeared during the procedure, the cortical SEP was abruptly lost. Return to near the baseline SEP pattern occurred in about 20 minutes.

Conclusions

Our preliminary data indicate that BAEP and SEP recording during surgical operations in the region of the cerebellopontine angle is a reliable method for monitoring brainstem function. Evoked potential alterations following mechanical traction or compression of nervous tissue reverted to normal in all cases and no neurological signs of brainstem function impairment developed postoperatively.

An interesting point in intraoperative electrophysiological monitoring was the dissociation between somatosensory and acoustic evoked response changes which we observed during dissection of a large neurinoma of the hypoglossal nerve. In this case, possible damage to brainstem structures would not have been detected by isolated recording of BAEPs.

Therefore, it appears that the combined recording of both SEPs and BAEPs may improve the sensitivity of the electrophysiological brainstem monitoring during operations in the posterior fossa.

References

1. Grundy BL (1982) Monitoring of sensory evoked potentials during neurosurgical operations: methods and applications. Neurosurgery 2: 556–575
2. Grundy BL, Jannetta PJ, Procopio PT, Lina A, Boston JR, Doyle E (1982) Intraoperative monitoring of brainstem auditory evoked potentials. J Neurosurg 57: 674–681
3. Jewett DL, Williston JS (1971) Auditory-evoked far fields averaged from scalp of humans. Brain 94: 681–696
4. Little JR, Lesser RP, Lueders H, Furlan AJ (1983) Brainstem auditory evoked potentials in posterior circulation surgery. Neurosurgery 12: 496–502
5. Piatt JH, Radtke RA, Erwin CW (1985) Limitations of brainstem auditory evoked potentials for intraoperative monitoring during a posterior fossa operation: case report and technical note. Neurosurgery 16: 818–821
6. Raudzens PA, Shetter AG (1982) Intraoperative monitoring of brainstem auditory evoked potentials. J Neurosurg 57: 341–348
7. Starr A, Hamilton AE (1976) Correlation between confirmed sites of neurological lesions and abnormalities of farfield auditory brainstem responses. Electroencephalogr Clin Neurophysiol 41: 595–608
8. Stockard JJ, Rossiter VS (1977) Clinical and pathologic correlates of brainstem auditory response abnormalities. Neurology 27: 316–325

Electrophysiological Monitoring of Intraoperative Cerebral Hypoperfusion States

L. Lutzemberger, G. Parenti, G. Tusini

Institute of Neurosurgery, University of Pisa (Italy)

Introduction

Critical low levels of blood flow and oxygen supply may induce irreversible structural damage of nervous tissue. Ischemic injury follows the impairment of membrane electrical properties[1, 2, 3, 11] which may be easily detected by the recording of spontaneous or evoked cerebral electrical activity[4, 5, 7, 15, 18]. For this reason electroencephalography (EEG) and somatosensory evoked potentials (SEPs) have been used to reveal possible functional consequences of low perfusion states[8, 9, 10, 12, 14, 15, 16, 17].

In carotid endarterectomy (CEA), the artery must be clamped during reconstructive surgery. A low flow state may also occur in cerebrovascular procedures if the temporary occlusion of a major cerebral vessel is performed during the dissection and clipping of a vascular malformation.

Intraoperative EEG and SEP recording during CEA and cerebrovascular procedures can reveal possible cerebral functional alterations when still reversible. During carotid occlusion, an increase in systemic arterial blood pressure (BP) or the placement of a bypass shunt is generally sufficient to normalize cerebral perfusion and electrophysiological recordings. In the case of temporary occlusion of a cerebral artery, the development of SEP alterations is an index of inadequate cerebral blood flow (CBF) and indicates the need for clip removal.

It is worth stressing that anesthetics such as halothane or isoflurane may have a considerable effect on both spontaneous and evoked electrical activity[6, 13, 19]. For this reason the maintenance of a stable level of anesthesia is important for the comparison of the electrophysiological recordings before and during vessel occlusion.

Methods

Two-channel EEGs and SEPs were monitored during 27 CEAs and 27 cerebrovascular procedures (24 aneurysms and 3 A-V malformations).

Spontaneous cerebral electrical activity was recorded by a processed EEG monitor (Interspec Neurotrac). Two symmetrical channels from biparietal electrodes were acquired. Two-second periods of EEG activity (from 0 to 3.0 Hz) were analyzed using a fast Fourier transform and displayed as a plot of frequency (x-axis) against power (y-axis). Successive epochs of EEG were then displayed as a compressed spectral array (CSA). SEPs following median nerve stimulation at the wrist were recorded from the second cervical spine and from the scalp over the contralateral somatosensory area, using a frontal reference and a bandpass of 5 to 800 Hz. Square waves of 0.3 msec duration were delivered to the stimulating electrodes at a rate of 5/sec. Stimulus intensity was three times twitch threshold. 256 repetitions were averaged. Induction of anesthesia was performed with sodium thiopental 5 mg/kg. The patient was intubated using succinylcholine and artificially ventilated with a mixture of 40% oxygen and 60% nitrous oxide. Pancuronium bromide in appropriate doses was used as muscle relaxant. Isoflurane was given as the main anesthetic agent in concentrations ranging from 0.3 to 1%. In all cases blood gas analysis was carried out at frequent intervals. The arterial pCO_2 was maintained at 30–35 mmHg.

In 5 aneurysms a temporary clip was applied to a major vessel (Table 1), three to the middle cerebral artery (MCA) and two to the proximal anterior cerebral artery (ACA). Approximately 10 minutes before vessel occlusion, bolus doses of thiopental were given until burst suppression was seen on CSA recording. Additional barbiturate was then administered by bolus injection as necessary to maintain burst suppression. During barbiturate infusion, isoflurane concentration was reduced.

Table 1

Cerebrovascular operations monitored by SEPs		Temporary vessel occlusion (barbiturate infusion, EEG burst suppression)
ICA aneurysm	6	—
A Com A aneurysm	9	2
MCA aneurysm	6	3
ACA aneurysm	3	—
A-V malformations	3	—
		CCT (msec) Mean ± SD n = 5
Before operation		5.9 ± 0.8
Induction of anesthesia		6.4 ± 0.6
Barbiturate infusion		7.3 ± 1.0
Vessel occlusion		7.4 ± 1.1
End of operation		6.7 ± 0.7

The parameters utilized during intraoperative monitoring were:

1. interhemispheric symmetry of CSA;

2. central conduction time (CCT) defined as the difference between poststimulus latencies of N 20 and N 14;

3. amplitude and latency of late SEP components.

SEPs were recorded before operation, after the induction of anesthesia and continuously through the surgical procedure. During CEA, the evoked responses used as "control" were the ones recorded immediately before carotid clamping. In cerebrovascular procedures SEPs monitored during vessel occlusion were compared with those recorded after barbiturate administration.

A stable level of anesthesia, achieved by a constant concentration of anesthetic gas before and after vessel occlusion, was monitored by CSA of the normal hemisphere. Likewise a constant degree of EEG burst suppression was monitored by CSA recording.

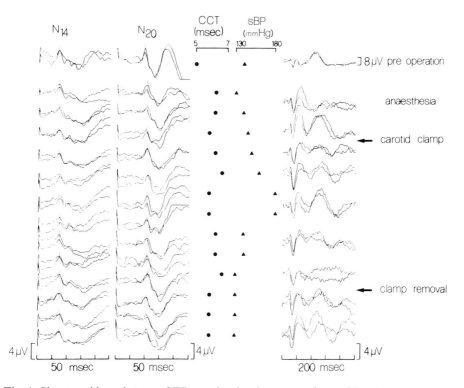

Fig. 1. Short and long latency SEP monitoring in a case of carotid endarterectomy. After carotid clamping, the latency lengthening of N 20 and the amplitude attenuation of the evoked potentials are reversed by raising systolic BP up to 180 mmHg. The same SEP morphology and CCT values achieved during carotid occlusion at a BP of 180 mmHg are obtained, after clamp removal, at a systolic of 130 mmHg

Results

During the majority of CEA procedures (20/27 cases) with an average carotid clamping time of about 60 minutes, no electrophysiological alterations were recorded.

In one patient, during carotid dissection but before clamping, bilateral EEG alterations, increased CCT and changes in long latency SEP were seen when systolic BP fell from 150 to 105 mmHg. Elevation of the BP was immediately followed by normalization of EEG and SEP.

In another case a progressive increase of the CCT (to 1.5 msec above baseline) and a morphological alteration of the N 20-P 22 complex developed during carotid clamping and persisted after clamp removal. No neurological deficits were present at the end of the operation.

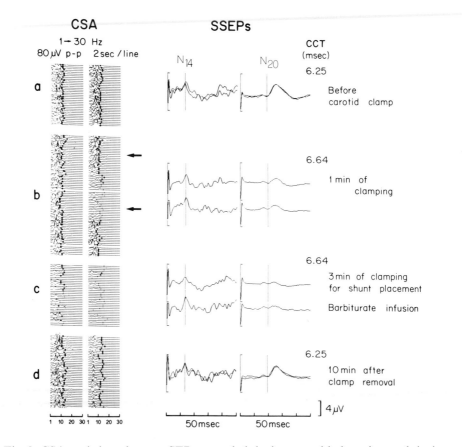

Fig. 2. CSA and short latency SEPs recorded during carotid clamping and during shunt placement under barbiturate infusion (see EEG burst suppression in (c). The upper and lower arrows indicate clamp placement and clamp removal respectively. Systolic BP: 160 mmHg

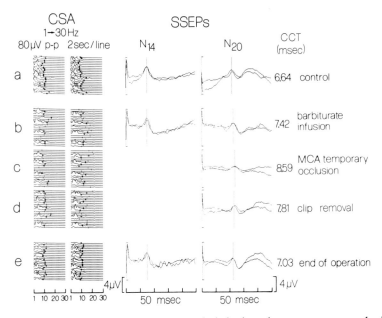

Fig. 3. CSA and short latency SEPs recorded during the temporary occlusion of a MCA under barbiturate infusion (thiopental 300 mg). SEPs displayed in (c) were recorded about 3 minutes after clip placement and in (d) SEP recording was performed 4 minutes after clip removal. Systolic BP: 110 mmHg. CSA recorded in (b, c), and (d) shows a constant level of EEG burst suppression

In three patients SEP changes developed without any EEG modification after clamp placement and were reversed by raising systemic BP. In Fig. 1 the relationship between systolic BP and CCT during temporary occlusion of the carotid artery and after clamp removal is shown. Two different levels of systemic pressure were necessary during and after carotid occlusion to record comparable SEPs.

Two of the 27 patients required a shunt on the basis of EEG and SEP changes. In one of these patients (Fig. 2) clear EEG and SEP alterations developed about 20 sec after carotid clamping at a systolic BP of 160 mmHg. Shunt placement under barbiturate protection was followed by normalization of both EEG and SEP signals. In the other case, despite shunt placement, permanent neurological deficits occurred postoperatively as a consequence of severe arterial hypotension following acute intraoperative myocardial infarction. In 5 aneurysm cases in which a temporary clip was applied to a branch of the MCA (3 cases) or to one proximal ACA (2 cases) with an occlusion time of 3 to 16 minutes, barbiturate infusion at doses necessary to induce EEG burst suppression did not obliterate the N 20 wave of the SEP. In these cases, CCT was the best indicator of cerebral function. In 4 patients, CCT during the entire period of vessel occlusion did not differ from that measured after EEG burst suppression induced by thiopental. In one patient (Fig. 3), the ischemic effect of MCA temporary occlusion under barbiturate treatment was shown by the increased latency and the attenuated amplitude of early SEPs. CCT was reduced to earlier values promptly after the clip was removed.

Discussion

SEP monitoring during CEA and cerebrovascular procedures is a reliable method for evaluating cerebral function even during barbiturate administration titrated to EEG burst suppression. Only one of the patients monitored had neurological deficits at the end of the operation, in agreement with persistent electrophysiological alterations recorded intraoperatively. In patients undergoing surgery for CEA, functional ischemic damages related to systemic arterial hypotension may occur even before carotid clamping. Intraoperative electrophysiological monitoring allowed an early correction of the low flow state.

SEP alterations developed during carotid clamping in 6 cases. It is important to stress that in 3 of these patients electrophysiological normalization was easily obtained by raising systemic BP. Thus shunt placement with its possible complications was avoided.

The depression of spontaneous electrical activity secondary to barbiturate administration did not prevent evaluation of cerebral function by continuous monitoring of CCT during the temporary occlusion of a major cerebral vessel. It must be stressed, however, that SEP recording using stimuli from the posterior tibial nerve would be a more adequate method to assess possible ischemia in the territory of the ACA during its temporary occlusion. Ischemia in this area might not be detected in SEPs elicited by stimulation of the median nerve.

Intraoperative monitoring of CEA and cerebrovascular surgery was performed by the simultaneous recording of both SEPs and EEG, the latter displayed as CSA. CSA monitoring is less sensitive than SEP monitoring; in 4 of the 6 cases in which SEP changes occurred during carotid clamping, no CSA interhemispheric asymmetries were recorded. Moreover during EEG burst suppression following barbiturate treatment, CSA monitoring cannot be utilized to reveal possible interhemispheric differences. Nevertheless, in our experience CSA recording is a useful technique in intraoperative monitoring; it is a means of controlling the stability of the anesthesia and it allows real time monitoring of cerebral function by immediately detecting signs of ischemic functional damage (Fig. 2).

Hence, it seems that the combination of SEP and CSA recording can improve intraoperative monitoring through a more complete electrophysiological evaluation of the functional cerebral state than is provided by either technique alone.

References

1. Astrup J (1982) Energy-requiring cell functions in the ischemic brain. Their critical supply and possible inhibition in protective therapy. J Neurosurg 56: 482–497

2. Astrup J, Moller Sorensen P, Rahbek Sorensen H (1981) Oxygen and glucose consumption related to Na_+—K_+ transport in the canine brain. Stroke 12: 726–730

3. Astrup J, Siesjo BK, Symon L (1981) Thresholds in cerebral ischemia. The ischemic penumbra. Stroke 12: 723–725

4. Branston NM, Strong AJ, Symon L (1977) Extracellular potassium activity, evoked potentials and tissue blood flow. Relationships during progressive ischemia in baboon cerebral cortex. J Neurol Sci 32: 305–321

5. Branston NM, Symon L, Crockard HA, Pasztor E (1974) Relationship between the cortical evoked potential and local cortical blood flow following acute middle cerebral artery occlusion in the baboon. Exp Neurol 45: 195–208

6. Clark DL, Rosner BS (1973) Neurophysiologic effect of general anesthetics. I. The electroencephalogram and sensory evoked response in man. Anesthesiology 38: 564–579

7. Cusick JF, Myklebust JB (1985) The relationship of somatosensory evoked potentials and cerebral blood flow. In: Cerebral revascularization for stroke. Thieme-Stratton Inc, New York, pp 160–165

8. Ducati A, Cenzato M, Landi A, Sironi VA, Massei R, Beretta L, Prati R, Bortolani E, Trazzi R (1985) Somatosensory evoked potentials and electroretinography compared with EEG during carotid endarterectomy. 8th International Congress of Neurological Surgery, Toronto

9. Grundy BL (1982) Monitoring of sensory evoked potentials during neurosurgical operations: methods and applications. Neurosurgery 11: 556–575

10. Grundy BL, Nelson PB, Lina A, Heros RC (1982) Monitoring of cortical somatosensory evoked potentials to determine the safety of sacrificing the anterior cerebral artery. Neurosurgery 11: 64–67

11. Heiss WD, Hayakawa T, Waltz AG (1976) Cortical neuronal function during ischemia. Effects of occlusion of one middle cerebral on single-unit activity in cats. Arch Neurol 33: 813–820

12. Markand ON, Dillay RS, Moorthy SS, Warren C Jr (1984) Monitoring of somatosensory evoked responses during carotid endarterectomy. Arch Neurol 41: 375–378

13. Mc Pherson RW, Mahla M, Johnson R, Traystam RJ (1985) Effects of enflurane, isoflurane and nitrous oxide on somatosensory evoked potentials during fentanyl anesthesia. Anesthesiology 62: 626–633

14. Raudzens PA, Spetzler RF, Carter LP, Wilkinson E (1985) Cerebral electrical activity during low flow states. In: Cerebral revascularization for stroke. Thieme-Stratton Inc, New York, pp 187–196

15. Sharbrough FW, Messick JM Jr, Sundt TM Jr (1973) Correlation of continuous electroencephalograms with cerebral blood flow measurements during carotid endarterectomy. Stroke 4: 674–683

16. Sundt TM Jr, Houser OW, Sharbrough FW, Messick JM Jr (1977) Carotid endarterectomy: results, complications and monitoring techniques. Advances in Neurology 16: 97–119
17. Symon L, Wang AD, Costa e Silva IE, Gentili F (1984) Perioperative use of somatosensory evoked responses in aneurysm surgery. J Neurosurg 60: 269–275
18. Umbach C, Heiss WD, Traupe H (1981) Effect of graded ischemia on functional coupling and components of somatosensory evoked potentials. J Cereb Blood Flow Metab 1: S 198–S 199
19. Wang AD, Costa e Silva IE, Symon L, Jewkes D (1985) The effects of halothane on somatosensory and flash visual evoked potentials during operations. Neurol Res 7: 58–62

SEP and EEG Monitoring During Carotid Surgery

E. Fava, A. Ducati*, E. Bortolani**, M. Cenzato*, A. Landi*,
D. Ghilardi***, R. Trazzi***

CNR Institute of Muscle Physiology c/o * Institute of Neurosurgery, ** Institute of General and Cardiovascular Surgery and *** II Chair of Anesthesiology, University of Milano (Italy)

Introduction

A great deal of arterial pathology responsible for ischemic alterations of the brain is amenable today to surgical treatment, particularly when it involves the extracranial carotid arteries. Perioperative neurologic complications still range from 1 to 10%[1], resulting from a variety of causes: impaired cerebral perfusion during carotid occlusion, distal embolization of atheromatous fragments, carotid artery thrombosis, and reperfusion injury[2]. Several methods have been developed by anesthesiologists and surgeons focusing on the early detection of reduced cerebral function during the carotid surgery and prevention of permanent brain injury.

In this study, somatosensory evoked potentials (SEPs) elicited by median nerve stimulation and eight channels of the electroencephalogram (EEG) were recorded in patients requiring thromboendarterectomies (TEA) of the common or internal carotid arteries and in a few patients receiving carotid-subclavian artery bypasses, to correct subclavian steal phenomena.

Both SEPs and EEG rely on the adequacy of cerebral perfusion. Focal EEG slowing has always been considered the first sign of cerebral impairment. SEPs, on the other hand, provide more easily quantifiable indices of cortical and subcortical activity, and their alterations develop at a rate that is faster at greater levels of ischemia[3].

Our aim was to correlate intraoperative SEP recordings with EEG alterations and with the occurrence of perioperative neurologic complications. We monitored both short and long latency evoked responses, not only during the period of carotid occlusion, but during the entire surgical procedure.

Clinical Materials and Methods

During the 24 months before this conference, 45 patients selected for carotid endarterectomy because of transient ischemic attacks and 4 patients requiring carotid-subclavian artery bypass grafting for subclavian steal syndrome were operated upon under general anesthesia. The ages of the patients ranged from 54 to 78 years (mean 62.8 years). Each patient was subjected to Doppler evaluation and intravenous digital subtraction angiography or selective four-vessel angiography of the cerebral arteries. Of the 45 patients requiring carotid endarterectomy, 32 had unilateral stenosis, 10 had bilateral stenosis, and 3 had contralateral occlusion.

After induction with a short-acting barbiturate, anesthesia was maintained by neuroleptic and analgesic drugs and the patients were slightly hyperventilated with 60% nitrous oxide in oxygen, with moderate doses of isoflurane (0.4–1.5%) when required. Arterial blood pressure was monitored continuously by means of a Statham pressure transducer attached to a catheter inserted into the radial artery, and it was kept at a patient's usual level.

Esophageal temperature was in the range 35.5–36 °C.

Somatosensory evoked potentials (SEPs) were recorded by means of commercial systems (Amplaid MK 10 and Amplaid MK 15). Recordings were obtained on the day before surgery, after the induction of anesthesia, each 5 min during vessel preparation, each 1–2 min during the carotid clamping, and again each 5 min after unclamping until the surgery was over.

For preoperative assessment and at the beginning of the surgery, SEPs were obtained from both right and left parietal areas upon stimulation of the contralateral median nerves. During the critical phases of the operations, SEPs were usually monitored only from the cortex ipsilateral to the carotid artery that was to be clamped, but if any change was detected, responses from the contralateral parietal cortex were obtained to compare the SEPs on the two sides. The stimulus was delivered by a constant current stimulator to the median nerve at the wrist by means of subdermal needle electrodes 3 cm apart with the cathode proximal. Stimulus duration was 0.2 msec, the intensity was adjusted to a value exceeding three times the threshold for thumb twitch before administration of muscle relaxants (about 20 mA), and stimulation frequency was 1–4 Hz. Recordings were obtained by using subdermal platinum electrodes from parietal (C 3'-C 4') and upper cervical (SC 2) locations, both referred to the FpZ position[4]. With such a montage the cervical responses (N 13), the short latency cortical SEP (N 20) and the long latency cortical waves were recorded. For N 13 and N 20 recording, the analysis time was 30 msec, filter bandwidth 10–2,500 Hz, and stimulation rate 4 Hz; 300–500 repetitions were averaged.

For long latency cortical SEP the analysis time was 200 msec, filter band-width 1–200 Hz, and stimulation rate 1 Hz; 100 sweeps were averaged. An automatic artifact rejection device was employed, but the unprocessed electroencephalographic activity was continuously observed. The morphology of the entire cortical responses, N 20 peak latency, N 13–N 20 central conduction time (CCT)[5], and N 20–P 22 peak-to-peak amplitude recorded during the period of carotid clamping were compared serially and also with intraoperative preclamp recordings.

The EEG was recorded during the entire operation by using an eight channel bipolar montage. Nine stainless steel needle electrodes were placed symmetrically over both frontal, central, parietal and occipital regions, the ground being on the nasion.

Results

A trial occlusion of the internal and common carotid arteries (mean duration 87 sec) was always performed in order to assess the need for a temporary indwelling shunt. We never observed focal EEG flattening or complete loss of the cortical evoked responses after test carotid clamping. However, 39 of 49 patients (nearly 80%) showed a change of some size in either or both of the neurophysiological tests. Altogether, we found that 30 patients had a minimal, usually bilateral, EEG change and 30 patients had at least one SEP modification. Only 18 patients had both abnormalities (Fig. 1).

SEP changes were never a mere prolongation of the CCT during trial occlusion: the increase in CCT up to 3.2 msec was observed only in association with an amplitude reduction of the SEP primary component to a mean value of 2/3 of the baseline amplitude. It is interesting to note

Neurophysiological changes during trial occlusion

(39 patients)

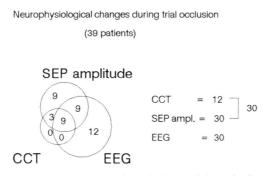

Fig. 1. SEP and EEG changes occurring during trial occlusion of the common and internal carotid arteries. *CCT* prolongation of the somatosensory central conduction time; *SEP ampl* amplitude reduction of the whole cortical response; *EEG* any alteration in amplitude or frequency on the electroencephalographic recording

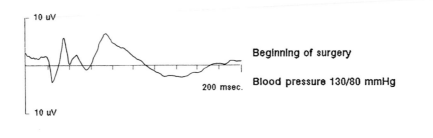

LEFT INTERNAL CAROTID ARTERY ENDARTERECTOMY

Cortical SEPs upon right median nerve stimulation

Patient B.G. — Jan. 22, 1986

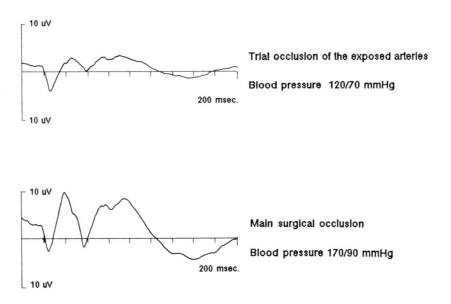

Fig. 2. Effect of drug induced hypertension on reversing SEP modification occurring in patient B.G. just after trial clamping of the carotid. Negativity is
displayed as downward deflection

that 9 patients not showing any change in CCT had EEG slowing and a
significant reduction in SEP amplitude.

All the changes observed during trial carotid occlusion were substantially reversible with deliberate hypertension (Fig. 2), possibly as a consequence of improved collateral circulation. The changes in neurophys-

Neurophysiological changes during main occlusion

(46 patients)

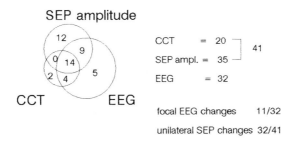

Fig. 3. SEP and EEG changes occurring during the main carotid occlusion for the reparative phase of the surgery. Abbreviations as in Fig. 1

iological parameters were not judged so severe as to require the use of a temporary shunt, because shunting has its own complications (for example, see ref.[6]).

Carotid occlusion for the reparative phase of the surgery ranged from 11 to 37 min in duration (mean 22 min) and was carried out under moderate hypertension. A change in neurophysiological parameters was observed in 46 of 49 patients. 41 showed SEP changes of some kind and 32 had a modified EEG. 27 patients exhibited both SEP and EEG abnormalities (Fig. 3).

Focal EEG slowing was present in 11 of 32 patients, and unilateral SEP changes were observed in 32 of 41 patients. A mere CCT prolongation was present in only 2 patients, while, among the other 18 cases with an increased CCT, 4 were associated with a slowed EEG (2 focal) and 14 with both a slowed EEG (9 focal) and a significantly reduced SEP amplitude (below 2/3 of baseline trace amplitude). CCT maximal prolongation was 3.2 msec; absolute values for CCT were less than 9.0 msec in all cases but one and persisted as long as 15 minutes.

A single patient had a CCT of 9.2 msec associated with reduction in N 20–P 22 amplitude to 70% of baseline, with complete flattening of late waves and a very slight focal EEG slowing. These changes persisted for 20 minutes. In this specific case, stump pressure was also recorded and was always above 70 torr. Conjunctival oxygen tension was always above 50 torr. This patient awoke with a motor defect and one hour after surgery he was comatose (Fig. 4).

Discussion

The most dreaded complication associated with carotid surgery is the development of a stroke or the progression of a preexisting neurological

PATIENT T.W. (JAN. 13, 86) – RIGHT INTERNAL CAROTID ENDARTERECTOMY

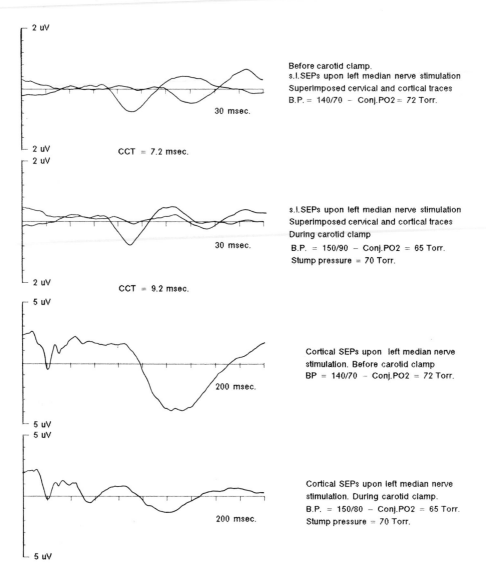

Before carotid clamp.
s.l.SEPs upon left median nerve stimulation
Superimposed cervical and cortical traces
B.P. = 140/70 – Conj.PO2 = 72 Torr.

CCT = 7.2 msec.

s.l.SEPs upon left median nerve stimulation
Superimposed cervical and cortical traces
During carotid clamp
B.P. = 150/90 – Conj.PO2 = 65 Torr.
Stump pressure = 70 Torr.

CCT = 9.2 msec.

Cortical SEPs upon left median nerve
stimulation. Before carotid clamp
BP = 140/70 – Conj.PO2 = 72 Torr.

Cortical SEPs upon left median nerve
stimulation. During carotid clamp.
B.P. = 150/80 – Conj.PO2 = 65 Torr.
Stump pressure = 70 Torr.

Fig. 4. SEP alterations occurring in the only patient who developed a perioperative complication. Note that CCT absolute value is abnormal even before the carotid occlusion. Negativity is displayed as downward deflection

deficit. Routine use of a temporary shunt may partly overcome the need for intraoperative assessment of cerebral function in patients operated upon under general anesthesia, but the use of a shunt has its own complications: intimal damage, embolization of atheromatous fragments, and interference with surgical procedure. Moreover, Prioleau *et al.*[6] reported a similar incidence of intraoperative strokes in shunted and non-shunted cases in a large series of patients and concluded that routine monitoring by stump pressure or EEG might help pick out patients that could theoretically benefit from a shunt. In the absence of clear indications, the use of a shunt does not seem warranted; the risks outweigh the benefits. Measurement of stump pressure is technically simple, but the range of critical pressure has not yet been firmly established. Continuous EEG monitoring has been the most extensively used monitoring technique, but there are technical difficulties and the EEG is highly sensitive to systemic factors such as depth of anesthesia, drugs, and hyper- and hypocapnia.

SEPs have been shown by many authors to be reliable indicators of central nervous system function in conditions of experimental brain ischemia[3, 7]. Moreover, cortical responses evoked by median nerve stimulation are assumed to be generated in the somatic sensory areas, supplied by the middle cerebral artery, where a great risk of ischemic injury is expected in case of carotid occlusion[8]; far field potentials reflect electrical conduction in the whole somatosensory pathway. On this basis, SEPs have been employed for several years in monitoring cerebrovascular surgery. Many reports in the literature agree that irreversible obliteration of the somatosensory evoked response is associated with new postoperative neurological deficits (see ref.[1] and[9]).

Although we never observed the disappearance of the SEP, we recorded many minor SEP changes during occlusion of the carotid artery.

In our series, only three patients showed no SEP change during carotid clamping. The most frequent alterations observed during carotid occlusion were a reduction of the late waves and/or of N 20–P 22 amplitude. In only 11 cases was this pattern of change followed by unilateral EEG slowing. In all the other patients the SEP changes were followed by bilateral slowing of the EEG.

Two main conclusions seem appropriate: late waves and N 20–P 22 amplitudes usually diminish 1–2 min before EEG alterations are seen; these may be the most sensitive indices of brain malfunction. We found that induced hypertension, usually not exceeding 30% of the habitual level for each patient, was in most cases sufficient to restore the SEP waveform.

It seems possible to infer that SEP recording is not only more sensitive than EEG in detecting a cerebral ischemia, but more specific as well. In fact, the only patient who had a postoperative neurological complication showed a significant change in SEPs, while the EEG was only minimally slowed during carotid occlusion. We actually observed more severe changes in other patients in this series who did not show any new postoperative neurological dysfunction.

Prolongation of CCT up to 3.2 msec, even if associated with N 20–P 22 amplitude reduction of 80% was not followed by clinical worsening. It appears that due consideration must be given to the absolute value reached by the CCT, and to the time course of this change, as well as to the extent of CCT prolongation. In fact, the only patient in this series with neurological deterioration after operation showed a CCT of 9.2 msec; as its baseline value was 7.2 msec, the prolongation in this case was only 2 msec.

In conclusion, we agree that quantitative tolerance limits for acceptable degrees of intraoperative SEP changes are lacking. However, this does not detract from the utility of SEP monitoring in carotid surgery, where the method appears to be both sensitive and specific.

A pattern of SEP change that seems to indicate serious risk for the patient is a prolongation of the CCT to longer than 9 msec, associated with a significant reduction of evoked response amplitude. The presence of unilateral EEG slowing is, in this context, not essential.

The goal of intraoperative monitoring is to minimize the risk of permanent brain damage, and this can be accomplished in a highly sensitive and reproducible way with SEP monitoring. The superimposition of sequential records, requiring only a few seconds for each record, facilitates observation of the evolution of any observed change as well as the effects of measures taken to protect the brain. It is evident that any change in the evoked responses must be communicated to the surgeon and anesthesiologist so that it can be evaluated in light of what is happening to the patient from multiple points of view; only such a global assessment can make monitoring useful for decision making.

References

1. Russ W, Fraedrich G, Hehrlein FW, Hempelmann G (1985) Intraoperative somatosensory evoked potentials as a prognostic factor of neurologic state after carotid endarterectomy. Thorac Cardiovasc Surg 33: 392–396
2. Steed DL, Peitzmann AB, Grundy BL, Webster MW (1982) Causes of stroke in carotid endarterectomy. Surgery 92: 634–641
3. Branston NM, Symon L, Crockard HA, Pasztor E (1974) Relationship between the cortical evoked potential and local cortical blood flow following acute middle cerebral artery occlusion in the baboon. Exp Neurol 45: 195–208
4. Jasper HH (1958) The ten-twenty electrode system of the international federation. Electroencephalogr Clin Neurophysiol 10: 371–375
5. Hume AL, Cant BR (1978) Conduction time in central somatosensory pathways in man. Electroencephalogr Clin Neurophysiol 45: 361–375
6. Prioleau WH Jr, Aiken AF, Hairston P (1977) Carotid endarterectomy: neurologic complications as related to surgical techniques. Ann Surg 185: 678–683
7. Hargadine JR, Branston NM, Symon L (1980) Central conduction time in primate brain ischemia: a study in baboons. Stroke 11: 637–642

8. Grundy BL, Sanderson AC, Webster MW, Richey ET, Procopio P, Karanjia PN (1981) Hemiparesis following carotid endarterectomy. Anesthesiology 55: 462–466
9. Grundy BL (1985) Intraoperative applications of evoked responses. In: Owen JH, Davis H (eds) Evoked potential testing. Grune & Stratton Inc, Orlando, U.S.A., pp 159–212

Intraoperative Monitoring of Scalp-recorded SEPs During Carotid Endarterectomy

M. Caramia, F. Zarola, G. L. Gigli, F. Lavaroni, P. M. Rossini

Laboratorio di Neurofisiologia clinica, Dipartimento di Sanità pubblica,
Il Università di Roma (Italy)

Introduction

Carotid endarterectomy (CEA) represents one elective treatment for selected patients suffering from stenotic or ulcerative carotid lesions.

This surgical procedure poses risks of possible acute brain ischemia either due to progressive decrements of cerebral blood flow (CBF) during carotid occlusion, or secondary to embolization, mostly occurring when a temporary shunt is inserted[26, 32].

CEA outcome may be improved by early intraoperative detection of cerebral dysfunction prior to transient or permanent injury in the territory supplied by distal branches of the middle cerebral artery (MCA) which perfuses large portions of the sensorimotor cortex.

Short latency somatosensory evoked potentials (SEPs), recorded from cervical and scalp electrodes in response to median nerve (MN) stimulation, represent a noninvasive technique particularly indicated for exploring the function of afferent somatosensory pathways, from the periphery to the sensory cortex, via spinal and intracranial relays[9, 29].

By means of such a method, one might define the approximate subcortical and cortical level of altered signal propagation along the central somatosensory pathways due to transient ischemia in the most distal regions of the MCA.

In this study, we evaluated the modifications of cortical SEP components observed at precentral and postcentral recording sites and correlated them with postoperative neurological sequelae as well as with carotid stump pressures.

Patients and Methods

Forty CEAs, carried out in 37 patients (28 males, 9 females; mean age 62.5 years, range 38–78 years) were monitored after individual informed consent.

Clinical and ancillary examinations were consistent with the diagnosis of insufficient CBF in the area of the carotid artery (25 right, 15 left), due to ulcers or stenoses of different degrees.

The Department of Vascular Surgery considering these patients at particularly high risk because of their ages and clinical histories, requested SEP monitoring.

Intraoperatively CBF was indirectly evaluated before arteriotomy by measuring stump pressure[20]. According to Hunter *et al.* (1982), 50 mmHg is considered a safe level of stump pressure for prolonged carotid clamping; values between 25 and 50 mmHg are considered at risk, and those below 25 mmHg require shunting.

The stump index (stump pressure/systolic BP) was also evaluated and considered to indicate shunting when below 20.

SEP recordings were performed using Ag/AgCl disk electrodes glued to the skin with collodion. Exploring electrodes were placed on the ipsilateral (Ci) and contralateral (Cc) parietal scalp sites overlying the primary somatosensory cortex, and the contralateral motor (Cc') cortex for the hand. The terms ipsilateral and contralateral refer to the scalp ipsilateral and contralateral to the side of MN stimulation. The Ci and Cc electrodes were 2 cm caudal and the Cc' electrodes 2 cm rostral to the C 3 and C 4 positions of the International 10–20 system. An electrode was also placed on the rostral-most cervical spine (CV 2) to monitor the stability of the incoming volley entering the brainstem. A common noncephalic reference electrode was positioned on the contralateral shoulder. Contralateral-to-ipsilateral scalp derivations were also utilized to cancel out subcortical components and enhance cortical activity.

All the recordings were performed using filters with a bandpass of 16–1,600 Hz (-12 dB/oct.), an analysis time of 50 msec poststimulus, and a sampling rate of 10,000 Hz per channel (OTE Basis EPM). Constant current rectangular stimuli (15–45 mA, 0.1–0.15 msec duration) with an intensity sufficient induce a slight thumb twitch before curarization were delivered at a rate of 9–11 Hz, through a surface stimulating probe firmly positioned over the MN at the wrist contralateral to the affected carotid. A large belt ground was placed 7–8 cm proximal to the stimulating cathode.

Final traces were averages of 200–300 artifact-free responses and were replicated every 40 sec, stored on floppy disks for further off-line analysis, and printed on paper.

The following peak latencies, interpeak intervals and amplitudes were evaluated: cervical N 13 latency and amplitude, latencies of the scalp N 20 and P 25, N 13–N 20 central conduction time (CCT), and N 20–N 25 peak-to-peak amplitude. The latency and peak-to-peak amplitude of the P 22–N 30 complex recorded from the precentral electrode was also evaluated.

According to data gathered in the initial part of the study, amplitude decrements of the cortical waves were considered significant only when below 50% of the pre-clamping values, in the presence of steady peripheral and spinal input as shown by the amplitude of the Cv 2 response and of the subcortical P 9, P 11, P 13, P 14 components.

Latency delays causing a CCT prolongation of at least 1 msec, with respect to the pre-clamping values, were considered abnormal.

Table 1. *List of Patients Who Did Not Present Alterations of SEPs as Defined in the Text*

Case	Sex	Age	Side	Stump	I.S.	Shunt	Seq.
1	m	72	r	40	36	n	N.D.
2	f	62	r	75	42	n	N.D.
3	m	58	r	48	33	n	N.D.
4	m	65	r	48	34	n	N.D.
5	f	58	r	98	42	n	N.D.
6	m	60	l	63	35	n	N.D.
7	m	65	r	43	43	n	N.D.
8	m	65	r	40	26	n	N.D.
9	m	62	l	45	24	n	N.D.
10	m	71	r	33	31	n	N.D.
11	m	41	l	60	40	n	N.D.
12	m	65	r	55	37	n	N.D.
13	m	64	r	40	38	n	N.D.
14	m	58	r	69	48	n	N.D.
15	m	79	r	76	45	n	N.D.
16	f	64	r	55	27	n	N.D.
17	m	75	l	70	37	n	N.D.
18	m	72	l	82	50	n	N.D.
19	m	61	r	19	20	y	N.D.
20	m	51	r	63	41	n	N.D.
21	m	64	r	47	38	n	N.D.
22	m	54	l	26	30	n	N.D.
23	f	46	l	41	37	n	N.D.
24	m	65	l	33	29	y	N.D.
25	m	68	r	40	33	n	N.D.
26	f	63	r	35	19	n	N.D.
27	m	57	r	72	50	n	N.D.
28	f	38	r	70	45	n	N.D.
29	f	70	r	40	31	y	N.D.
30	m	66	r	80	50	n	N.D.

I.S. = Index of Stump = Stump/Systolic pressure × 100.
Seq. = Neurological complications on awakening.
N.D. = No Deficit.

Amplitude and latency variations were considered significant only when seen in 3 successive averages.

The intraoperative monitoring protocol included several SEP recordings before curarization, then additional recordings before carotid clamping and during measurement of stump pressure, as well as during and after clamping of the carotid artery. More than 100 trials were stored and evaluated for each patient. Throughout the operation arterial blood pressure (BP), heart rate (HR), and arterial blood gases were monitored.

Neurological status was assessed in the days preceding the operation and immediately after awakening from anesthesia. If any deterioration of the neurological status was found, follow-up of neurological examination was performed at 3–4 day intervals for two weeks.

Results

SEP monitoring showed no significant modification in 30 of the 40 examined CEAs. In 3 cases a temporary shunt was positioned during the

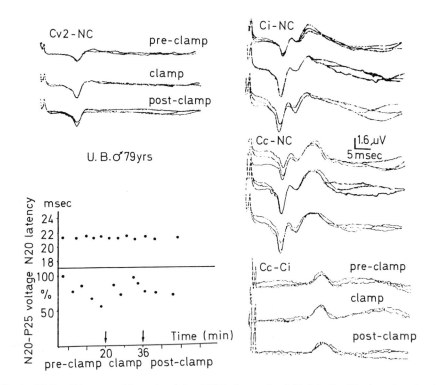

Fig. 1. U. B., 74-year-old male right CEA (case 5 of Table 2). Notice that both the subcortical and cortical components of SEPs remained unmodified during the different phases of the surgical procedure. At postoperative examination, this patient had no neurological sequelae

Table 2. List of Patients Presenting Alterations of SEPs as Defined in the Text

Case	Sex	Age	Side	Stump	I.S.	Shunt	Seq.	SEPs Alterations (Abrupt = A; Gradual = G; Recovered = R; Not Recovered = NR)					
								N20 latency		N20–P25 amplitude		CCT N13–N20	
1	m	59	l	83	52	N	P.D.	A	NR	A	NR	A	NR
2	m	71	l	89	78	N	T.D.	A	NR	A	NR	A	NR
3	m	58	r	27	17	Y	T.D.	G	NR	G	NR	A	NR
4	m	80	l	40	19	Y	T.D.	G	R	G	NR	G	R
5	m	74	r	54	27	N	N.D.	G	R	G	NR	G	R
6	f	62	l	25	25	Y	N.D.	G	R	G	R	G	R
7	f	64	l	40	26	N	N.D.	G	R	G	R	G	R
8	f	54	l(ECA)	ICA occlusion		N	N.D.	G	R	G	R	G	R
9	m	67	r	52	37	Y	N.D.	G	R	G	R	G	R
10	m	59	l	40	20	Y	N.D.	G	R	G	R	G	R

I.S. = Index of Stump = Stump/Systolic Pressure × 100.
Seq. = Neurological Complications on Awakening.
P.D. = Permanent Deficit.
T.D. = Transient Deficit (Complete recovery before the end of the 15-day follow up).
N.D. = No Deficit.

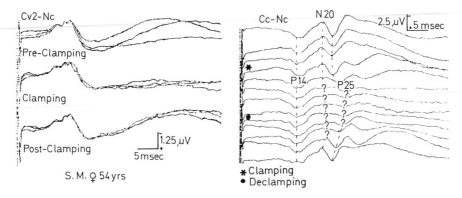

Fig. 2. S. M., 54-year-old female (case 8 of Table 2). A left CEA was performed on a stenotic ECA in presence of a totally occluded ICA. In spite of stable spinal and subcortical components of SEPs, about 3 min after ECA clamping a gradual and progressive amplitude decrease and latency delay affected the parietal N 20–P 25 complex. This provoked a speeding up of the surgical procedure. After declamping the cortical complex progressively reacquired the original characteristics in a time interval of about 17 min. On awakening the patient did not present any worsening of the preoperative neurological examination

entire course of the surgical intervention because of low stump pressures. Transient SEP amplitude decrements, affecting both subcortical and cortical components, were observed in association with falls in BP, but none of these patients had neurological sequelae (Table 1 and Fig. 1).

In the remaining CEAs, significant abnormalities of scalp SEPs were seen after carotid clamping (Table 2). Changes consisted of delayed N 20–P 25 wave latencies and decreased amplitudes of the N 20–P 25 complex. Such alterations completely recovered before awakening from anesthesia in 5 of 10 patients (Fig. 2). In 3 patients the recovery was spontaneous, while in the other 2 it occurred after a shunting device was placed. None of these 5 patients developed neurological sequelae. In 3 of the 5 remaining cases, abnormalities of scalp SEPs were still present at the end of the surgical intervention, showing transient or stabilized signs of CNS damage (Figs. 3, 4, and 5). In the fourth patient a 50% decrease in N 20–P 25 amplitude was still present at the end of intervention, without neurological deficits on awakening from anesthesia. However, during the course of the following day this patient became aphasic and hemiparetic.

In the last patient a progressive flattening of the N 20–P 25 complex was seen immediately after the carotid clamping and only the N 20 wave recovered after declamping (Fig. 6). On awakening, right hemiparesis and mild motor aphasia were present; the symptoms disappeared in 3 days.

We found that SEP abnormalities appeared in a gradual and progressive

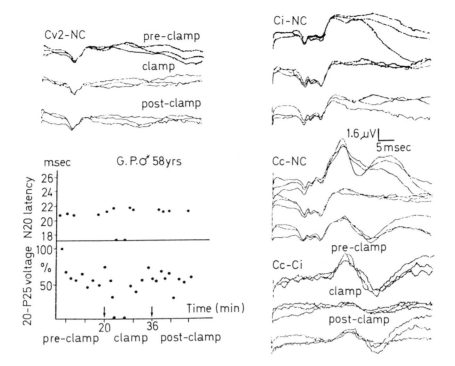

Fig. 3. G. P., 58-year-old male (case 3 of Table 2). In this patient, who had a low stump pressure (27 mmHg) during right CEA, a progressive flattening of the cortical response was observed, while the subcortical events were unchanged. The amplitude decrement of the N 20–P 25 complex was preceded by a gradual, progressive prolongation of its latency which began 60–90 sec after carotid clamping. Despite positioning of a shunt device, when the carotid was reopened this cortical complex reappeared with a significantly decreased amplitude and delayed latency, never regaining its preclamping values. After awakening from anesthesia, this patient complained of severe contralateral hypaesthesia for all sensory modalities. He completely recovered in a few days

fashion 3–6 min after carotid clamping (Fig. 3) in all but 2 cases (Figs. 4 and 5) in which they were briskly precipitated by carotid occlusion. In 2 patients we observed complete disappearance of precentral components along with alterations of the parietal waveforms. After shunt placement the parietal complex partially regained its preclamping values, while the precentral P 22 was still absent and only reappeared after reopening of the carotid artery.

These findings seem to support the hypothesis of separate generators for short latency SEPs facing each other at pre- and postcentral recording sites[8, 15, 25].

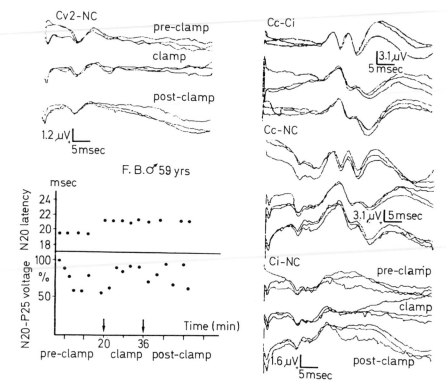

Fig. 4. F. B., 59-year-old male, left CEA (case 1 of Table 2). Immediately after clamping, despite steady subcortical responses, this patient had an abrupt delay of N 20 peak latency (about 2 msec) coupled to a fluctuating amplitude which never decayed below 50% of preclamping values even though the following intermediate latency waves completely disappeared. These modifications persisted during the entire clamping period and after restoration of circulation. Stump pressure was 83 mmHg. At neurological examination after awakening, this patient had motor aphasia and contralateral hemiparesis and did not recover

Discussion

The incidence of short term neurological complications following CEA ranges from 2 to 4% because of ischemia due to inadequate collateral vascularization during carotid clamping or due to embolization[7, 32]. The incidence is even higher in those patients in whom a temporary shunt is required. In the past 17 years several monitoring techniques for evaluating the brain functionality and the adequacy of collateral CBF have been attempted, including continuous electroencephalography (EEG), evaluation of regional CBF, measurement of carotid stump pressure, and measurement of jugular venous oxygen saturation. All these have served to give only indirect documentation; but they do not reliably reflect cerebral

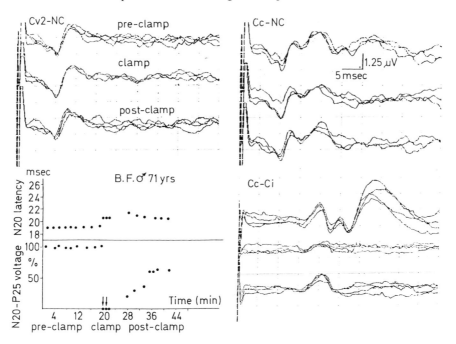

Fig. 5. B. F., 71-year-old male, left CEA (case 2 of Table 2). The N 20–P 25 complex and the following cortical waves entirely disappeared shortly after carotid clamping, even though stump pressure was 90 mmHg. The surgeon immediately declamped the carotid artery, and interrupted CEA. Despite this, and despite barbiturate administration, the SEPs did not return to baseline values. Ten minutes after carotid reopening, only a delayed N 20 of depressed amplitude reappeared. Postoperative neurological examination showed a moderate right-sided hemiparesis with a mixed aphasia. Neurological deficits gradually and almost completely recovered, but the patient died of intercurrent complications 3 days later

function and perfusion because of the influences exerted on them by various factors such as the level of anesthesia and other neurodepressant drugs, the length of the evaluating procedure, or the intrinsic variability of the measured parameters. Stump pressure in particular does not provide information on the patency of the more distal vessels of the MCA territory. Moreover, this index can be obtained only before and during endarterectomy. Even though experimental studies in animals showed a close relationship between CBF and the spontaneous cortical electrical activity recorded by the EEG, this technique does not directly reflect the function of subcortical structures. Also EEG is considerably affected by factors such as the concentrations of anesthetic agents and fluctuations of BP[2]. In contrast experimental and clinical studies have shown that early SEP components are little affected by anesthetic drugs and only briefly influenced by large systolic pressure variations. SEPs to peripheral nerve stimulation

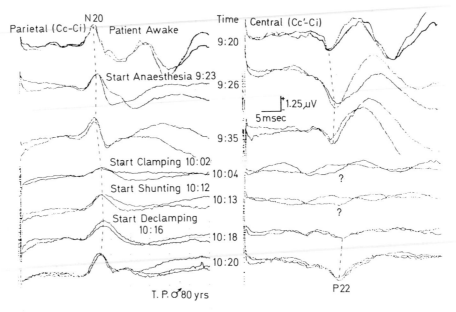

N 20
Parietal (Cc-Ci)   Patient Awake   Time   Central (Cc'-Ci)
                                                          9:20

                          Start Anaesthesia 9:23
                                                          9:26

                                                               ⊥ 1.25 μV
                                                                5 msec

                                                          9:35

                          Start Clamping 10:02
                                                          10:04   ?

                          Start Shunting 10:12
                                                          10:13
                                                                    ?
                          Start Declamping
                          10:16
                                                          10:18

                                                          10:20

                          T. P. ♂ 80 yrs   P 22

Fig. 6. T. P., 80-year-old male, left CEA (case 4 of Table 2). Progressive and gradual delay of latency and decay of amplitude of the central posterior N 20–P 25 complex were seen after clamping. Wave N 20 recovered the preclamping characteristics partially after shunting and further after declamping. However, the P 25 and following waves remained undetectable. The central anterior P 22 (right) showed an evolution independent from the one of the central parietal N 20–P 25 complex. On awakening, this patient presented a mild motor aphasia with right hemiparesis, and gradually recovered in the following 3 days

are highly stable and reproducible responses, faithfully reflecting the function of the afferent pathways from the peripheral nerve to the related cortical structures.

On this theoretical framework it seems that SEPs might be extensively utilized for real time monitoring of brain function during CEA, representing a reliable indirect index of CBF.

Our results concerning the CEAs monitored with multichannel SEP lead to the following conclusions:

– stable SEPs with normal CCTs throughout CEA procedure were never followed by new neurological deficits;

– transient or permanent neurological sequelae were not predicted by stump pressure values, but were always preceded by increases in intracranial CCT (P 14–N 20) of more than 1 msec and by persistent (> 3 min) amplitude decreases of the N 20–P 25 complex below 50% of the preclamping values. One patient with low stump pressure who presented unmodified SEPs did not develop neurological deficits despite not receiving a shunt.

On the contrary, good stump pressure values in 2 patients were associated with sudden development of SEP abnormalities and neurological complications;

— the simultaneous recording of SEP components generated outside the area of the carotid artery and cortical SEPs generated inside the area of the carotid artery permitted exclusion of "false" amplitude decrements secondary to technical factors such as decreased stimulation intensity, which, when occurring, both groups of waves affect simultaneously. On the other hand, changes due to carotid clamping showed selective alterations of cortical components while subcortical components were almost unaffected.

There seems to be a high correlation between the incidence of postoperative neurological complications and the rapidity of SEP deterioration after carotid clamping. Our observations indicate that those SEP modifications seen immediately after carotid clamping, presumably reflecting embolization in the MCA territory (Figs. 4 and 5) were invariably coupled to neurological sequelae. In contrast, when SEP changes appeared gradually, with progressive increases in latency and declines in amplitude, possibly related to deficient collateral vascularization, SEPs spontaneously recovered without any complication in 5 of 8 cases (cases 6–10 of Table 1).

The most important contribution of multichannel SEP monitoring seems to be provision of real-time information on the function of the cerebral structures. More series of CEAs are needed to better define the priority between stump-pressure values and significant SEP modifications in establishing when a shunt should be positioned.

References

1. Astrup J, Symon L, Branston NM, Lassen NA (1977) Cortical evoked potential and extracellular K^+ and H^+ at critical levels of brain ischemia. Stroke 8: 51–101
2. Baker JD, Gluecklich B, Watson CW, Marcus E, Kamat V, Callow AD (1975) An evaluation of electroencephalographic monitoring for carotid study. Surgery 78: 787–794
3. Branston NM, Symon L, Crockard HA, Pasztor E (1974) Relationship between the cortical evoked potential and local cortical blood flow following acute middle cerebral artery occlusion in the baboon. Exp Neurol 45: 195–208
4. Brunko E, Zegers de Beyl B (1986) Prognostic value of early cortical somatosensory evoked potentials after resuscitation from cardiac arrest. Electroencephalogr Clin Neurophysiol, in press
5. Chiappa KH (1983) Evoked potentials in clinical medicine. Raven Press, New York, pp 251–324
6. Chiappa KH, Burke SR, Young RR (1979) Results of electroencephalographic monitoring during 367 carotid endarterectomies. Use of a dedicated minicomputer. Stroke 10: 381–388

7. Connolly JE, Kwaan JH, Stemmer EA (1977) Improved results with carotid endarterectomy. Ann Surg 186: 334–342
8. Desmedt JE, Bourguet M (1985) Color imaging of parietal and frontal somatosensory potential fields evoked by stimulation of median and posterior tibial nerve in man. Electroencephalogr Clin Neurophysiol 62: 1–17
9. Desmedt JE, Cheron G (1980) Central somatosensory conduction in man: neural generators and interpeak latencies of the far-field components recorded from neck and right or left scalp and earlobes. Electroencephalogr Clin Neurophysiol 50: 382–403
10. Heiss WD, Waltz AG, Hayakawa T (1975) Neuronal function and local blood flow during experimental cerebral ischemia. In: Harper AM, Jennet WG, Miller JD, Rowan JO (eds) Blood flow and metabolism in the brain. Churchill Livingstone, Edinburgh, pp 27–28
11. Hobson RW, Wright CB, Sublett JW, Fedde CW, Rich NM (1974) Carotid artery back pressure and endarterectomy under regional anesthesia. Arch Surg 109: 682–687
12. Hossman KA, Schuier FJ (1980) Experimental brain infarcts in cats. I Pathophysiological observations. Stroke 11: 583–592
13. Hunter GC, Sieffert G, Malone JM, Moore WS (1982) The accuracy of carotid back pressure as an index for shunt requirements. A reappraisal. Stroke 13: 319–326
14. Markand ON, Dilley RS, Moorthy SS, Warren C (1984) Monitoring of somatosensory evoked responses during carotid endarterectomy. Arch Neurol 41: 375–378
15. Mauguiere F, Desmedt JE, Courjon J (1983 a) Astereognosis and dissociated loss of frontal and parietal components of somatosensory evoked potentials in hemispheric lesions: detailed correlation with clinical signs and computerized tomographic scanning. Brain 106: 271–311
16. Mauguiere F, Desmedt JE, Courjon J (1983 b) Neural generators of N 18 and P 14 far-field somatosensory evoked potentials in patients with lesions of thalamus or thalamocortical radiations. Electroencephalogr Clin Neurophysiol 56: 283–292
17. Mauguiere F, Ibanez V (1985) The dissociation of early SEP components in lesions of the cervico-medullary junction: a cue for routine interpretation of abnormal cervical responses to median nerve stimulation. Electroencephalogr Clin Neurophysiol 62: 406–420
18. Meneghetti G, De Riu GP, Saia A, Giaretta D, Ballotta E (1984) Continuous intraoperative EEG monitoring during carotid surgery. Eur Neurol 28: 82–88
19. Meyer KL, Dempsey RJ, Roy MW, Donaldson DL (1985) Somatosensory evoked potentials as a measure of experimental cerebral ischemia. J Neurosurg 62: 269–275
20. Moore WS, Hall AD (1969) Carotid artery back pressure. A test of cerebral tolerance to temporary carotid occlusion. Arch Surg 99: 702–710
21. Murphy F, Maccubin DA (1965) Carotid endarterectomy: a long-term follow-up study. J Neurosurg 23: 156–168

22. Ojemann RG, Crowell RM, Robertson GH, Fisher CM (1975) Surgical treatment of extracranial carotid occlusive disease. Clin Neurosurg 22: 214–263

23. Perez-Borja C, Meyer JS (1985) Electroencephalographic monitoring during reconstructive surgery of the neck vessels. Electroencephalogr Clin Neurophysiol 18: 162–169

24. Rossini PM, Di Stefano E, Stanzione P (1985) Nerve impulse propagation along central and peripheral fast conducting motor and sensory pathways in man. Electroencephalogr Clin Neurophysiol 60: 320–334

25. Rossini PM, Gigli GL, Marciani MG, Zarola F, Caramia M (1987) Noninvasive evaluation of input-output characteristics of sensorimotor cerebral areas in healthy humans. Electroencephalogr Clin Neurophysiol 68: 88–100

26. Sacquegna T, D'addato M, Baldrati A, Cortelli P, Lamieri C, Merlo Pich E, Vitacchiano G, Pedrini L (1986) Longterm prognosis after carotid endarterectomy. Eur Neurol 25: 36–39

27. Sato M, Pawlik G, Umbach C, Heiss WD (1984) Comparative studies of regional CNS blood flow and evoked potentials in the cat. Stroke 15: 97–101

28. Symon L, Hargadine J, Zawirski M, Branston N (1979) Central conduction time as a index of ischemia in subarachnoid hemorrhage. J Neurol Sci 44: 95–103

29. Symon L, Wang AD (1986) Somatosensory evoked potentials: their clinical utility in patients with aneurysmal subarachnoid hemorrhage. In: Cracco RQ, Bodis-Wollner I (eds) Evoked potentials. Frontiers of clinical neuroscience, vol 3. AR Liss, New York, pp 390–401

30. Symon L, Wang AD, Costa e Silva IE, Gentili F (1984) Perioperative use of somatosensory evoked responses in aneurysm surgery. J Neurosurg 60: 269–275

31. Sundt TM, Sharbrough FW, Piepgras DG, Kearns DP, Massik JM, O'Fallon WM (1981) Correlation of cerebral blood flow and electroencephalographic changes during carotid endarterectomy. Mayo Clin Proc 56: 533–543

32. Thompson JE (1979) Complications of carotid endarterectomy and their prevention. World J Surg 3: 155–165

33. Thompson JE, Patman RD, Talkington CM (1978) Carotid surgery for cerebrovascular insufficiency. Curr Probl Surg 15: 1–68

34. Trojaborg W, Boysen G (1973) Relation between EEG regional cerebral blood and internal carotid artery pressure during carotid endarterectomy. Electroencephalogr Clin Neurophysiol 34: 61–69

35. Umbach C, Heiss WD, Traube H (1981) Effect of graved ischemia on functional coupling and components of somatosensory evoked potentials. J Cereb Blood Flow Metab 1: S 198–S 199

36. Waltz AG, Sundt TM, Michenfelder JD (1972) Cerebral blood flow during carotid endarterectomy. Circulation 45: 1091–1096

SEP Monitoring During Carotid Surgery

G. De Scisciolo*, A. Amantini*, O. Ronchi*, M. Bartelli,
A. Peduto**, C. Paci**, C. Pratesi***, A. Alessi***, F. Pinto*

* Institute of Neurology, ** Department of Anesthesiology and Intensive Care,
*** Institute of Vascular Surgery, University of Florence (Italy)

Introduction

In carotid endarterectomy (CEA) carotid arteries need to be clamped for reconstructive surgery. Monitoring methods available for determining the adequacy of collateral blood flow include continuous EEG recording[12, 14], determination of stump pressure[8], measurements of regional cerebral blood flow (CBF)[17] and the assessment of neurological function with regional anesthesia in the conscious patient[9].

Intraoperative monitoring of somatosensory evoked potentials (SEPs) is being used increasingly for assessing cerebral function during surgery on intra- and extracranial arteries[5, 9, 15].

The main advantages of SEP monitoring are: relative resistance to general anesthesia, localization of SEP generators in the sensory-motor cortex selectively supplied by carotid perfusion, close relationship between SEP changes and local CBF values.

From a group of patients undergoing CEA, intraoperative SEP recordings were obtained in order to analyze evoked bioelectrical activity during clamping and shunt insertion and to relate SEP findings to the postoperative neurological status.

Cases and Methods

Twenty-five patients (age range 41–74 years) with histories of transient ischemic attack (TIA) or reversible ischemic neurologic deficit (RIND) were studied, all of whom presented carotid lesions appropriate to their symptoms.

SEPs were recorded continuously during CEA in response to stimulation of the contralateral median nerve at the wrist. The recording electrodes were placed over the sixth cervical spinous process (Cv 6) referred to FZ, and on the specific somatosensory projection area of each side, using either FZ or shoulder reference. The nerve was stimulated at the rate of 5 per sec, with pulse duration of 0.1 msec and stimulus intensity adjusted to induce a visible muscle twitch. The evoked responses were amplified with a filter band-pass of 5 Hz-5 KHz (-12 dB); time base for analysis was 100 msec. Each trial usually consisted of 150 averaged responses which were stored on a floppy disc for off-line analysis. Absolute latencies and amplitudes of N 13, P 14, N 20, P 25, N 33, P 40 and central conduction time (CCT) were measured before, during and after anesthesia. General endotracheal anesthesia was induced in all patients with meperidine (1.5 mg/kg), thiopentone (5 mg/kg) and atropine (0.015 mg/kg) and then maintained with nitrous oxide 40% in oxygen and isoflurane 0.6–0.8%. Heart rate, arterial blood pressure, arterial PO_2 and PCO_2 and shunt pressure were monitored. Stump pressure was also determined at clamping in all cases. A shunt was routinely used during reconstructive surgery, and mean occlusion time for our patients was 5.5 min (range 3–9 min).

Results

Poststimulus latencies of cortical SEP components as well as CCT increased significantly during anesthesia; the subcortical components were not affected (Table 1).

All cortical waves measured in the awake patient, including N 33 and P 40, were also identified during stabilized anesthesia and could be monitored constantly (Fig. 1). In most patients SEP parameters did not change significantly during the main phases of surgery, particularly after carotid clamping and shunt application. A reduction of N 20–P 25 peak-to-peak amplitude was observed but it did not reach statistical significance (Table 2). In some cases there were temporary SEP alterations which were not related to clamping or shunting: these were due to hypoxia or to systemic hypotension and rapid correction of such conditions promptly restored normal responses.

Table 1. *Effect of Anesthesia on the Latency of SEP Components*

SEP component	No anesthesia	Anesthesia	$P <$
N 13	14.62 ± 1.28	15.08 ± 1.30	NS
N 20	20.59 ± 1.12	22.07 ± 1.27	0.001
N 33	34.82 ± 3.78	42.23 ± 4.85	0.001
CCT	6.25 ± 0.82	7.23 ± 0.93	0.005

Values are means $\pm$ standard deviations in msec.

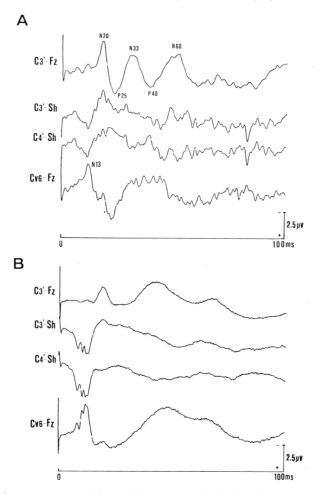

Fig. 1. SEPs in response to right median nerve stimulation in a patient before (A)
and during (B) stable anesthesia

Table 2. *Effects of Clamping on SEP Parameters*

SEP parameters	Pre-clamping	Post-clamping	p
N 13	14.67 ± 1.30	14.73 ± 1.35	NS
N 20	21.68 ± 1.28	21.95 ± 1.47	NS
N 33	41.98 ± 5.21	42.89 ± 5.24	NS
CCT	7.01 ± 0.67	7.22 ± 0.82	NS
N 20–P 25	2.07 ± 0.91	1.61 ± 0.87	NS

Values are means ± standard deviations in msec. Peak-to-peak amplitude N 20–
P 25 in uV.

Five of our 25 patients exhibited changes. Two of these showed an increase of CCT up to 9 msec during clamping and another exhibited a flattening of cortical waves except for N 20. SEPs were restored within a few minutes after shunt insertion for all three subjects. None of these patients had postoperative neurological deficits. In the other two cases we observed a complete intraoperative flattening of all cortical waves while the subcortical components remained unaffected. Both patients had post-operative neurological complications. For the first of these, angiography had shown an ulcerated stenosis of the left internal carotid with occlusion of the contralateral internal carotid. The CT scan and the preoperative neurological examination were normal. During surgery, one minute after clamping, this patient showed a progressive decrease in the amplitude of cortical waves, especially of the components following N 20. CCT remained unchanged. The stump pressure was 20 mmHg, suggesting inadequate collateral circulation. Shunt insertion restored a normal evoked response within a few minutes. Unfortunately, shunt thrombosis occurred, leading again to a progressive flattening of the cortical waves, including N 20. The components after N 20 were the first to be affected (Fig. 2). The recording with noncephalic reference showed during this time that the ipsi- and contralateral parietal responses became perfectly superimposable and that the negative ascending limb following P 14 was preserved (Fig. 3). The

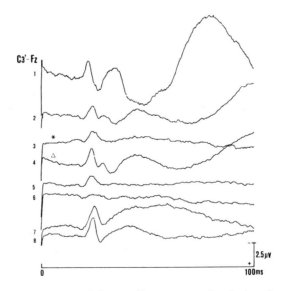

Fig. 2. SEPs in response to right median nerve stimulation in a patient with inadequate collateral circulation and right postoperative hemiparesis: (*1*) pre-anesthesia; (*2*) stabilized anesthesia; (*3*) clamping; (*4*) shunt application; (*5–6*) shunt thrombosis; (*7–8*) clamp removal

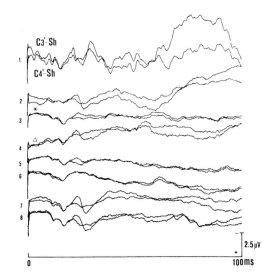

Fig. 3. SEP recording with non-cephalic reference obtained from the same patient at the same times as shown in Fig. 2. Traces of contra- and ipsilateral responses are superimposed

flattening of the traces lasted for almost 15 minutes, followed by an incomplete recovery characterized by a slight increase of the N 20 latency and an altered morphology of the cortical components. Postoperatively, the patient had a right hemiparesis which regressed partially in a matter of days.

In the second of our patients who showed a sudden disappearance of the cortical SEP, this flattening occurred immediately after shunt insertion. Shunt pressure was comparable to systemic pressure, suggesting an embolic ischemia. The patient had a postoperative monoparesis of the contralateral upper limp that lasted for six hours and then fully recovered. The day after surgery there was also a complete recovery of SEPs.

Discussion

Our data confirmed the marked sensitivity of SEPs to ischemia of the sensorimotor cortex as reported in previous animal and human studies[2, 11, 16]. Moreover, intraoperative SEP monitoring enabled us to promptly detect an episode of embolic ischemia.

Both amplitude and latency modification of SEPs occurred during different phases of surgery. However, no postoperative neurological deficit was seen unless there was a complete flattening of the waves, even if transitory.

Only by comparing ipsi- and contralateral parietal responses recorded with a noncephalic reference, can we correctly discriminate between cortical and subcortical SEP components[4]. We consider that such an electrode placement is essential for interpreting properly the flattening of early cortical waves, since the use of only the FZ reference might be misleading[10]. Our initial results, in agreement with those of previous reports[13, 16], suggest that amplitude changes in cortical SEP waves are closely associated with ischemia while latency changes are less reliable predictors of postoperative outcomes. It should be kept in mind that our observations were limited to a short period of carotid occlusion (less than 9 minutes) because intraluminal bypass shunts were routinely employed.

Inadequate collateral circulation and embolic ischemia produce characteristically different SEP modifications. In the former condition the flattening affects the latter cortical waves first and subsequently the early N 20. In the embolic ischemia, instead, there is an immediate and simultaneous disappearance of all cortical components. This finding emphasizes the importance of measuring the cortical waves following N 20, since these are the most sensitive to cortical ischemia. Unfortunately they are also very sensitive to anesthetic agents. However, the light anesthesia used in CEA permits constant monitoring of parietal N 33 and P 40 components. Later waves are too variable during surgery to serve as a reliable index of cerebral function for clinical purposes.

Controversy exists among surgeons about the usefulness of stump pressure for predicting tolerance to carotid occlusion. We observed no SEP changes at stump pressure values greater than 50 mmHg. For values between 20 and 40 mmHg SEPs were unchanged in some patients and altered in others. In fact, the critical pressure for the appearance of clinical deficits has so far not been firmly established[6, 7].

A discrepancy between the level of CBF which leads to the loss of the evoked responses and that which produces cerebral infarction has been fully demonstrated experimentally[1, 3] and this should be taken into account when evaluating intraoperative SEP changes.

We conclude that SEPs provide an excellent means of documenting and quantifying cerebral ischemia. Their prognostic value at present is limited, however, in that they fail to adequately predict postoperative neurological deficits.

References

1. Astrup J, Symon L, Branston NM, Lassen NA (1977) Cortical evoked potential and extracellular K^+ and H^+ at critical levels of brain ischemia. Stroke 8: 51–57
2. Branston NM, Symon L, Crockard HA, Pasztor F (1974) Relationship between the cortical evoked potential and local cortical blood flow following

acute middle cerebral artery occlusion in the baboon. Exp Neurol 45: 195–208

3. Branston NM, Strong AJ, Symon L (1977) Extracellular potassium activity, evoked potential and tissue blood flow. J Neurol Sci 32: 305–328

4. Desmedt JE, Cheron G (1980) Central somatosensory conduction in man: neural generator and interpeak latencies of the far-field components recorded from neck and right or left scalp and earlobes. Electroencephalogr Clin Neurophysiol 50: 382–403

5. Ducati A, Fava F, Landi A, Cenzato M, Bortoloni R, Trazzi R, Villani R (1985) SEPs and EEG monitoring during carotid endarterectomy. Electroencephalogr Clin Neurophysiol 61: 526–527

6. Hays RJ, Levinson SA, Wylie EJ (1972) Intraoperative measurement of carotid back pressure as a guide to operative management for carotid endoarteriectomy. Surgery 72: 953–960

7. Hobson RW, Wright LB, Sublett JW et al (1974) Carotid artery back pressure and arterectomy under regional anaesthesia. Arch Surg 109: 682–686

8. Hunter GC, Sieffert G, Malone JM, Moore WS (1982) The accuracy of carotid back pressure as an index for shunt requirements. Stroke 13: 319–326

9. Markand ON, Dilley RS, Moorthy JS, Warren CJ (1984) Monitoring of somatosensory evoked responses during carotid endoarteriectomy. Arch Neurol 41: 375–378

10. Mauguière F, Desmedt JE, Courjon J (1983) Astereognosis and dissociated loss of frontal or parietal components of somatosensory evoked potentials in hemispheric lesions. Brain 106: 271–311

11. Meyer RL, Dempsey RJ, Roy MW, Donaldson DL (1985) Somatosensory evoked potentials as a measure of experimental cerebral ischemia. J Neurosurg 62: 269–275

12. Mola N, Collice M, Levati A (1986) Continuous intraoperative electroencephalographic monitoring in carotid endarterectomy. Eur Neurol 25: 53–60

13. Ropper AH (1986) Evoked potentials in cerebral ischemia. Stroke 1: 3–5

14. Sharbrough FW, Messic FW, Messick JM, Sundt TM Jr (1974) Correlation of continuous electroencephalograms with cerebral blood flow measurement during carotid endarterectomy. Stroke 4: 674–683

15. Symon L, Wang AD, Costa e Silva IE, Gentili F (1984) Perioperative use of somatosensory evoked responses in aneurysm surgery. J Neurosurg 60: 269–275

16. Symon L, Wang J, Rosenstein J, Branston N, Tsutsui T (1985) Effect of brain ischemia on electrical activity in man. J Cereb Blood Flow Metab 5 [Suppl] 1: 837–838

17. Sundt TM Jr, Sharbrough FW, Pieppgras DG, Kearns TP, Messic JM Jr, O'Fallow W (1981) Correlation of cerebral blood flow and electroencephalographic changes during carotid endarterectomy. Mayo Clin Proc 56: 533–543

Intraoperative Monitoring During Extracorporeal Circulation

U. Ruberti, M. Cenzato*, A. Ducati*, E. Fava**, A. Landi*,
P. Giorgetti, R. Trazzi***

Institutes of General and Cardiovascular Surgery and * Neurosurgery, *** II Chair
of Anesthesiology, University of Milano, ** CNR Institute of Muscle Physiology,
c/o*, University of Milano (Italy)

Introduction

Modern anesthesiology has allowed surgeons to extend surgical treament
to areas once considered beyond approach. The technique of cardiopulmonary bypass, associated with hypothermia, makes it possible to maintain
a patient in extreme conditions; *i.e.,* the patient is kept alive for the whole
duration of a surgical procedure, with the heart at a standstill, with the
lungs not breathing, and with a mean arterial blood pressure of 40 mmHg
or below. The conditions necessary for heart surgery are allowed by hypothermia which lowers the metabolism of the body to facilitate survival in
these conditions. This is particularly important for the central nervous
system, where a temperature of 20–25 °C can effectively compensate for
the reduction of blood pressure and prevent neural damage. On the other
hand, it has been reported[2,5,10] that hypothermia may in itself cause neurologic injury. This view, however, is not shared by all authors. An adequate
balance is required between hypothermia (a factor offering some protection)
and hypotension (a potentially dangerous factor). Neural function should
therefore be monitored to verify whether, at specific levels of body temperature and of mean arterial pressure, the ability to respond to external
stimuli is preserved. Evoked potentials (EPs) have been useful and reliable
for this purpose. Within the central nervous system, the structure most
sensitive to ischemia is the cortex. For this reason, the study of the cortical
somatosensory response appears to be the best approach to the problem.
In the literature a few studies are reported[1,7,9] concerning evoked potential
monitoring during cardiopulmonary bypass. These papers mainly describe
subcortical and early cortical responses, the brainstem auditory evoked
potential (BAEP) and the short latency somatosensory evoked potential
(SSEP). It appeared that a detailed study of the entire cortical evoked

potential, including late waves, might help early identification of cortical dysfunction. Cortical SEPs are made up of a primary component, the N 20–P 25 complex, and late waves. The N 20–P 25 complex (often called simply N 20) is related to the arrival of the afferent sensory volley at the primary somatosensory cortex. All the later components are of cortical origin. The sensitivity of the primary component to anesthetic drugs is less than the sensitivity of later components, as these are mediated by a multisynaptic pathway. Our experience with intraoperative SEP monitoring during carotid surgery indicated that a change affecting late waves was the first sign of cortical ischemia, seen well before either prolongation of the N 20 latency or reduction of the SEP primary complex. In this study we tried to define the limits of EP changes seen when both body temperature (T) and blood pressure (BP) were modified in parallel.

Methods and Materials

We studied ten patients undergoing cardiac surgery. Ages ranged from 36 to 55 years. There were 9 males and 1 female; 2 were operated on for valvular insufficiency, 6 for aorto-coronary bypass, and 2 for multiple pathology (valvular and cardiovascular). All patients were neurologically normal before surgery, and none had a history of neurological deficits.

All the patients were premedicated two hours before surgery with atropine and morphine. General anesthesia was induced with a short-acting barbiturate, maintained with nitrous oxide and isoflurane, and supplemented as necessary with neuroleptoanalgesic drugs.

Muscle relaxants were used as well. Anesthetic levels were kept as constant as possible for the duration of the surgical procedures. After cannulation of a femoral artery and the right atrium, patients were gradually perfused with their own refrigerated blood. Finally the heart was arrested with cold cardioplegic solution and patients were supported by extracorporeal circulation only.

During the entire surgical procedure, esophageal and rectal temperatures, arterial blood pressure and the electrocardiogram (ECG) were continuously monitored. The lowest temperature reached was 20.4 °C, and the lowest blood pressure was 10 mmHg.

Evoked potentials were monitored by using a multimodality device, the Amplaid MK 10. Stainless steel needle electrodes were placed on the median nerve at the wrist for stimulation. Stimuli were electric shocks of 20 mA delivered to the nerve at a frequency of 1 or 4 pulses per second for cortical or short latency SEPs, respectively. Platinum subdermal needle electrodes were used for recording. Recording sites for SSEPs were Erb's point homolateral to the stimulus, the neck at the level of the second cervical vertebra (SC 2) and the parietal region contralateral to the stimulus (C 3′ or C 4′

according to the EEG International 10–20 System). Recording for cortical SEPs was from C3′ or C4′. The reference was always frontal (FpZ). Impedance of the electrodes was always below 5 KOhm. For SSEPs, analysis time was 30 msec and 500 sweeps were averaged with a filter bandwidth of 10–2500 Hz. For cortical SEPs, 100 sweeps were averaged with a 200 msec analysis time and a filter bandwidth of 1–200 Hz. Cortical SEPs were evaluated considering the morphology of the trace and the amplitude and the latency of the components, as described below. In all cases, the exploring electrode negativity was plotted as a downward deflection. Intraoperative recordings were collected at intervals ranging from 1 minute to 15 minutes depending on the surgical phases of the procedure, from the beginning to the end of anesthesia. Note was taken of the body temperature and blood pressure values at which each trace was collected.

The morphology, latency and amplitude of evoked potentials in the anesthetized patient differ from those recorded from the awake subject[6]. Control traces were therefore first obtained as soon as anesthesia was stable, using each patient as his own control. We examined the neurological status of the patient in the immediate postoperative period and when discharged from the hospital, to detect any possible neurological damage due to the surgical procedure.

For data analysis, six parameters of each cortical SEP trace were measured (Fig. 1): N 20 latency and amplitude, N 35 [the first negative wave of the late waves[4]] latency and amplitude, the total amplitude of the late waves, and, finally, the total number of peaks of the late waves.

Mean arterial blood pressure (MAP) was calculated as systolic pressure plus twice diastolic pressure, divided by 3. As far as amplitude is concerned, to obtain a homogeneous set of data each numeric parameter was normalized relative to the maximal value obtained in the specific patient during the surgical procedure. Then, in order to compare and to treat statistically all data from all patients, as a grand average, the value of each normalized parameter was transformed to its corresponding arcotangent value. This value was the one used in statistical analysis. To study the relative importance of body temperature and of blood pressure in affecting EP traces, the value of latency and of amplitude were separately tested against BP

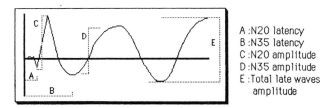

A :N20 latency
B :N35 latency
C :N20 amplitude
D :N35 amplitude
E :Total late waves
    amplitude

Fig. 1. Points of a typical cortical SEP on which measurements were based

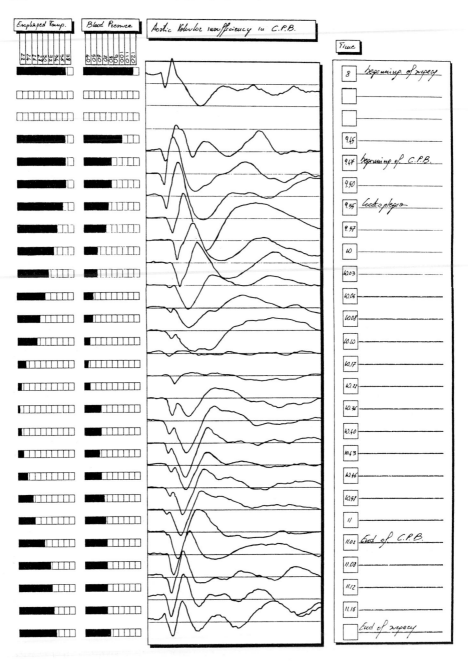

Fig. 2. Time course of esophageal temperature, blood pressure and cortical SEP traces during a surgical procedure for aortic valvular insufficiency. The correspondence among the three parameters during the entire surgical procedure is remarkable

and MAP levels, respectively, in single linear regression; afterwards, a multiple linear regression analysis was performed.

Results

Figure 2 shows the typical sequence of cortical SEP recordings obtained during surgery. The parallel decrease of MAP and of body temperature (T) causes a progressive increase of wave latencies and a decrease of amplitudes. With further decrease of MAP and T, N 35 and later waves become

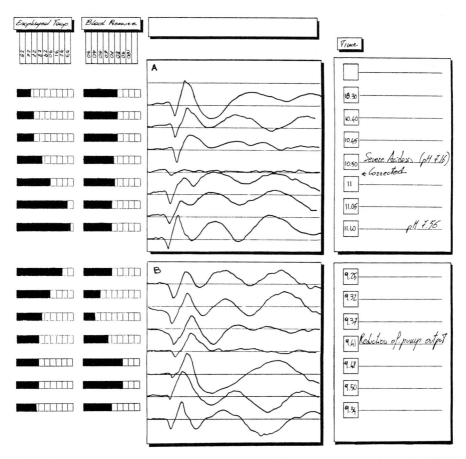

Fig. 3. Time course of esophageal temperature, blood pressure and cortical SEP traces during two single surgical procedures in which metabolic changes or reduction in pump output occurred. (A) Refers to the metabolic changes. At time 10.50 a severe acidosis occurred, with blood pressure unchanged and esophageal temperature increasing. Note the reduction in amplitude of the trace. (B) Refers to reduction of pump output (time 9.41). Esophageal temperature and blood pressure are in "safe" range

no longer visible, while N 20 is still evident, although delayed. The trace obtained at time 10.10 demonstrates that at the lowest values of MAP and T no cortically generated activity is any longer present; a small negativity persists on the cortical electrodes, but it must be of subcortical origin, as it always precedes the N 20 wave. Upon rewarming the patient, the cortical activity reappears, with progressively shorter latency and larger amplitude. This behavior was shared by all patients but one, who will be discussed below; in 9 patients, at temperatures of 22–25 °C and with a MAP of 30 torr, no cortical activity could be recorded for as long as 30 minutes. As all 9 had a normal neurological evaluation after surgery, the above described figures may be considered as safe tolerance limits for EP changes.

When the cortical activity was abnormal at higher levels of temperature and pressure, then it always appeared to be a significant surgical or anesthetic problem. For instance, the first sign of severe acidosis during rewarming of a patient was the sudden disappearances of all cortical activity (Fig. 3 A, trace at time 10.50); earlier absence of late waves signaled a critical reduction of the pump output, which was immediately corrected (Fig. 3 B, trace 9.41). To statistically analyze the combined effect of MAP and T on cortical evoked activity, we considered the grand average of all data derived from all patients (see Methods). Latency and amplitude changes of N 20 are shown in Fig. 4 (A, B). Confirming previous reports[8, 9], the effect of T on N 20 latency was striking; below 32 °C, a linear relationship existed between the two sets of values, with a high correlation ($r = -0.8392$). Little change was seen with variation in MAP ($r = -0.3478$). The amplitude of the N 20–P 25 complex appeared to be unchanged when MAP and T were above 55 torr and 32 °C, respectively. Below those values, the amplitude decreased. While the regression was not significant considering either MAP or T against N 20 amplitude, the multiple regression showed a high degree of correlation ($r = 0.95$). N 35 latency and amplitude (Fig. 5 A, B) behaved in a similar manner as N 20. The effect of T was manifest at a higher value (34–35 °C) and showed good correlation with latency ($r = -0.7539$). Moreover, at the same temperature, the mean amplitude of N 35 was much less than N 20 amplitude, confirming the observation made for the single patient in Fig. 2.

The point marked A in Figs. 4 and 5 deserves a detailed discussion. It refers to data from the last patient, who had an intraoperative aortic dissection that caused a prolonged drop in MAP when the temperature was still elevated. At a MAP of 44 torr and T of 34.5 °C, N 35 amplitude was near 0, and its latency was greater than 100 msec. The corresponding N 20 changes were definitely less striking. Two considerations may be drawn from this case, the only patient with severe postoperative neurological sequelae. First, N 35 was an earlier and more sensitive index of brain ischemia than N 20. Second, hypothermia actually did protect the brain from ischemic insults,

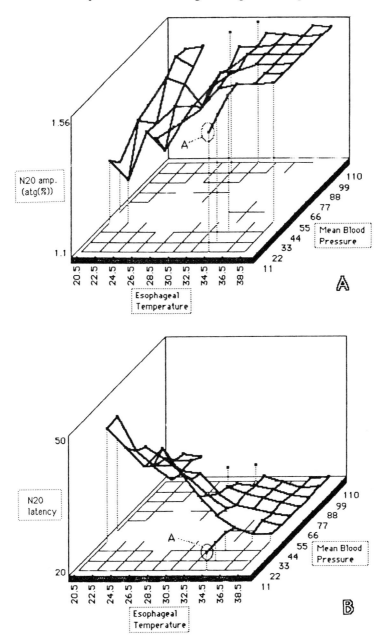

Fig. 4. (A) Trend of N 20 amplitude related to mean arterial blood pressure and esophageal temperature. Values for N 20 amplitude are not the actual values but the percent values, treated as described in the Method section in the text, with respect to the baseline value for any single patient. The point marked with *A* refers to data of the only patient who died. Note the drop in blood pressure. (B) Trend of absolute N 20 latency values plotted against mean arterial pressure and esophageal temperature

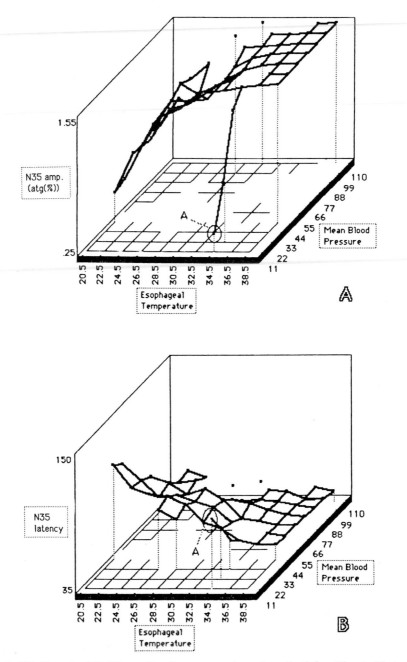

Fig. 5. (A) Trend of N 35 amplitude processed as described for Fig. 4. Note the fall in amplitude at the point marked with *A*. (B) Trend of N 35 peak latency plotted against mean arterial blood pressure and esophageal temperature. Note the increase in latency at the point marked with *A*

and within the explored value, did not cause injury. In fact, lower levels of MAP and of T were reached and maintained in all the other patients, without any neurological problem. Finally, the amplitude and morphology of longer latency waves did not show different behavior from N 35.

Discussion

The above data are in agreement with the work of Markand *et al.* and Hume *et al.*[7,9] concerning the increase of N 20 latency during hypothermia. The same effect was documented for N 35 and for later waves as well. In contrast with other reports, in which the blood pressure was kept constant, in our series a parallel reduction of MAP and of T was achieved. It appears that hypothermia can protect the brain from ischemia following a reduction of MAP well below the autoregulation range. The only patient in which a reduction of MAP was not accompanied by a parallel reduction of T presented with an immediate loss of cortical activity and suffered severe postoperative sequelae. An unprotected decrease in blood pressure was not the only cause of SEP change; similar modifications appeared as first signs of blood acidosis and of a fall in pump output. Acidosis may follow a sudden increase in metabolism, during rewarming of the patient, when tissue perfusion does not parallel the increase in temperature. A change in the patient's vascular resistance may, on the other hand, account for a reduction of the pump output with a consequent reduction of brain perfusion, an apparently adequate MAP notwithstanding. SEPs appear to be very sensitive to any potentially harmful factor, although with little or no specificity. From this point of view, the evaluation of N 35 and later waves seems to be more useful than the measurement of N 20 parameters. In fact, as N 35 changes are the first to appear, there is more time for the surgeon and for the anesthesiologist to identify the cause of the altered brain response and to treat it. EP alterations to be considered potentially dangerous are those falling outside the diagram showing averaged data of all patients. In addition, the disappearance of a previously seen wave, at lower values of MAP and T in a specific patient, is an index of cerebral dysfunction as well. The rationale for recording SEP cortical waves during heart surgery is therefore to give the surgeon and the anesthesiologist a further "warning signal", in order to increase the safety of patients.

References

1. Aren C, Badr G, Feddersen K, Radegran K (1985) Somatosensory evoked potentials and cerebral metabolism during cardiopulmonary bypass with special reference to hypotension induced by prostacyclin infusion. J Thorac Cardiovasc Surg 90: 73–79

2. Brunberg JA, Reilly EL, Doty DB (1974) Central nervous system consequences in infants of cardiac surgery using deep hypothermia and circulatory arrest. Circulation [Suppl] 11: 60–68

3. Coles JG, Taylor MJ, Pearce JM, Lowry NJ, Stewart DJ, Trusler GA, Williams WG (1984) Cerebral monitoring of somatosensory evoked potentials during profoundly hypothermic circulatory arrest. Circulation 70: 196–202

4. Colon EJ, de Weerd AW (1986) Long-latency somatosensory evoked potentials. J Clin Neurophysiol 3: 279–296

5. Egerton N, Egerton WS, Kay JH (1963) Neurologic changes following profound hypothermia. Ann Surg 157: 366–374

6. Grundy BL (1982) Monitoring of sensory evoked potentials during neurosurgical operations: methods and applications. Neurosurgery 11: 556–575

7. Hume AL, Durkin MA (1986) Central and spinal somatosensory conduction times during hypothermic cardiopulmonary bypass and some observations on the effects of Fentanyl and Isoflurane anesthesia. Electroencephalogr Clin Neurophysiol 65: 46–58

8. Kopf GS, Hume AL, Durkin MA, Hammond GL, Hashim SW, Geha AS (1985) Measurement of central somatosensory conduction time in patients undergoing cardiopulmonary bypass: an index of neurologic function. Am J Surg 149: 445–448

9. Markand OM, Warren CH, Moorthy SS, Stoelting RK, King RD (1984) Monitoring of multimodality evoked potentials during open heart surgery under hypothermia. Electroencephalogr Clin Neurophysiol 59: 432–440

10. Wright JS, Hicks RG, Newman DC (1979) Deep hypothermia arrest: observations on later development in children. J Thorac Cardiovasc Surg 77: 466–468

SEP Monitoring During Aortic Surgery

R. Trazzi*, E. Fava**, A. Ducati***, E. M. Bortolani****,
M. Cenzato***, A. Landi***, L. Seccia*

* II Chair of Anesthesiology, ** CNR Institute Muscle Physiology, c/o *** Institute of Neurosurgery, **** Institute of General and Cardiovascular Surgery, University of Milano (Italy)

Introduction

Surgical procedures requiring temporary occlusion of the descending aorta expose patients to the risk of ischemic injury to the spinal cord. The incidence of complete neurologic lesions complicating the resection of thoracic aortic aneurysms is reported as high as 24% of operated cases, with the greatest risk following operations for acute traumatic aortic rupture and elective resection of extensive thoraco-abdominal aortic lesions[2]. Neurological complications are less frequent following abdominal aortic aneurysm surgery; Szilagyi *et al.*[5] reported that the incidence of spinal cord damage was 0.25% in a series of more than three thousand operations. The necessity for ligation and exclusion of multiple intercostal and lumbar vessels during the course of operative repair of lesions, mainly in the thoracic and thoraco-abdominal aorta, may result in the permanent, though inadvertent, interruption of vessels critical for blood supply to the spinal cord. Paraplegia may result. Such catastrophic neurological complications have been, up to now, undetectable during the surgical procedure.

The blood supply to the spinal cord is highly variable. Preoperative angiographic identification of the critical vessels is rare. Furthermore, angiography is an invasive technique that may itself cause damage.

Numerous adjuncts, such as temporary shunt and bypass techniques, have been introduced by surgeons in attempts to improve distal aortic perfusion. However, these devices are ineffective in preventing spinal cord injury if, during the course of the surgery, vessels supplying the spinal cord are permanently interrupted or are inadequate to tolerate even the briefest aortic cross-clamping. Several cases are reported in the literature of spinal cord ischemia developing despite the intraoperative use of left atrial-femoral artery bypass or jump graft bypass techniques during surgery upon the thoracic aorta.

Even the time of aortic occlusion doesn't seem to be related to spinal cord injury in all cases[4].

In this study, we recorded cortical and spinal somatosensory-evoked potentials upon lower limb stimulation in a series of patients undergoing elective reparative surgery for lesions affecting the thoracic and abdominal aorta. SEPs were used for early detection of ischemic cord dysfunction during aortic occlusion.

Methods

SEPs were recorded during elective aortic operations performed for thoracic aneurysms, abdominal infrarenal aneurysms, aortoiliac occlusive diseases and femoral pseudoaneurysm. The surgical procedures for aneurysm repair were aneurysmectomy and Dacron graft replacement; for aortoiliac occlusive disease either endarterectomy or aortobifemoral Dacron graft replacement was carried out. The level of aortic cross-clamping was just below the left subclavian artery in thoracic lesions and infrarenal in surgery of the abdominal aorta.

Somatosensory-evoked responses were obtained by commercial system (Amplaid MK 10), using electrical stimulation of both posterior tibial nerves at the ankle or both common peroneal nerves just below the knee by means of a pair of a stainless steel subdermal needle electrodes, 3 cm apart, the cathode proximal. Impulse duration was 0.2 msec, intensity 20 mA, repetition rate 4 Hz. Both spinal and cortical SEPs were recorded with platinum needle subdermal electrodes, with impedance less than 5 Kohm each and interelectrode difference less than 2 Kohm. Analysis time was 100 msec, filtering bandwidth 10–2,500 Hz. We averaged 300–500 sweeps.

The spinal potential was recorded from L 3, with reference to T 12 or the iliac crest. Great attention was required in order to minimize the stimulus artifact in recording the lumbar response, so that the least disturbed recording arrangement was chosen in each patient. The latency of the major negative peak was taken as the reference time when the afferent volley enters the lower spinal cord through the dorsal roots. This allowed slowing in peripheral nerve conduction velocity, due to changes in limb temperature, to be largely ignored[1].

The cortical evoked potentials were recorded from the midline central area with a frontal reference. The amplitude of the whole cortical response and the peak latency of the first positive wave (P 37 from posterior tibial nerve stimulation at the ankle or P 27 from peroneal nerve stimulation at the knee) were measured.

Both spinal and cephalic responses were recorded on the day before surgery, after the induction of anesthesia, each 10 min during the vessel preparation, each 2 min during arterial occlusion, and each 5–8 min after unclamping until the end of the operation. A complete neurologic examination was performed on the day before surgery and as soon as the patients awoke after anesthesia. No patient had preoperative sensory or motor deficits.

Anesthesia was induced with a short-acting barbiturate and then maintained with narcotics, tranquilizers, and 60% nitrous oxide in oxygen. Moderate doses of isoflurane (0.4–1%) were added as necessary.

Results

We monitored more than 100 patients undergoing cardiovascular surgery. This presentation, however, deals only with a few patients operated upon for lesions of the thoracic and abdominal aorta who showed significant intraoperative changes in SEPs, elicited by lower limb stimulation.

Included in this report is the only patient with paraplegia following the repair of an abdominal aneurysm among the 72 cases operated upon during the last year. We also describe two subjects with bad outcomes of the 17 operated upon for thoracic aortic aneurysm.

Abdominal Aortic Surgery

When the infrarenal aorta and the iliac arteries were clamped, a change in SEPs was very common. The typical modification was a progressive prolongation in latency and a decrease in amplitude of the cortical response. Such changes occurred either immediately or at various intervals, up to 25 min after clamping.

Three patterns of change were apparent. First, the cortical response is absent while the lumbar spinogram is almost unchanged (Fig. 1); an ischemic spinal cord lesion may occur.

In the second case, the spinogram disappears while the cortical response maintains its usual morphology and shows only minor variations in latency. This pattern points to peripheral nerve ischemia. The response of the large peripheral nerve fibers, whose activity produces the surface-recorded lumbar spinogram, is abolished. Some fibers continue to transmit, however, perhaps in a desynchronized manner, and indeed the cortical response is present.

The third pattern of change is a parallel reduction and disappearance of both peripheral and cortical responses; there is no way to discriminate between nerve or spinal cord ischemic insult.

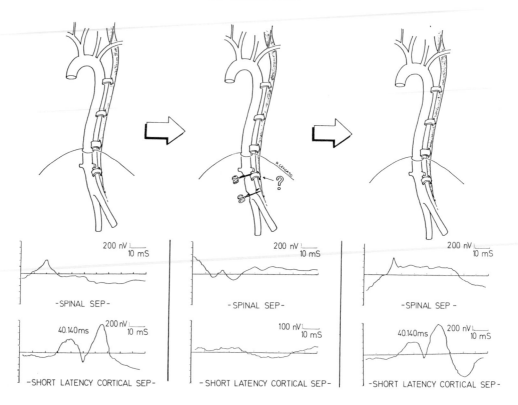

Fig. 1. Abdominal aortic surgery. In the upper part of the picture is a schematic drawing of the descending aorta and of the blood supply feeding the spinal cord. The small arrow with the question mark refers to the uncertain origin of the great radicular artery. In the lower part of the picture, lumbar and cortical records following posterior tibial nerve stimulation before, during and after occlusion of the abdominal aorta. Negativity upward for spinal SEP and downward for cortical
SEP

Independent of the combination of peripheral and central ischemic alterations, we observed that as long as the cephalic activity did not disappear for more than 30 minutes, the patient recovered without any complication.

A single patient presented with an absent cortical response for as long as 50 minutes. He continued to be unconscious to the end of the surgery and required mechanical ventilation for 24 hours. On the following day he was alert, but paraplegia with complete sensory loss was apparent. This severe complication cannot be ascribed with absolute certainty to an intraoperative cord ischemia, because the patient also developed an ischemic hepatic necrosis and an intestinal infarction. A multiple embolic episode, involving the spinal cord as well as the liver and intestine, cannot be ruled out.

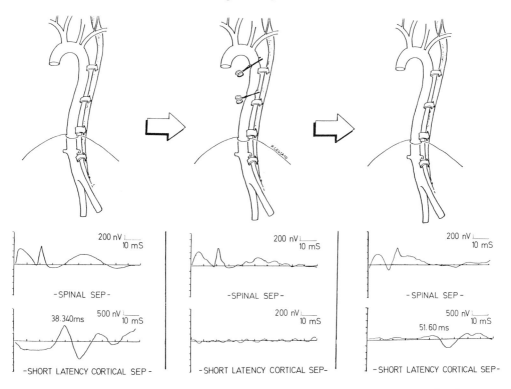

Fig. 2. Thoracic aortic surgery. Upper part as in Fig. 1. In the lower part, lumbar and cortical SEP following posterior tibial nerve stimulation before, during and after occlusion of the thoracic aorta. Polarity as in Fig. 1

However, the association of a long period of absent cortical SEPs with a severe postoperative neurological complication is to be considered with the utmost care.

Thoracic Aortic Surgery

Neurological complications with this approach are much more common than with operations on the abdominal aorta. In fact, 2 patients of the 17 operated upon had a bad outcome and one of them died. In the first patient (Fig. 2), a woman with an aneurysm, the cortical response disappeared 19 minutes after the thoracic aorta was clamped just below the origin of the left subclavian artery. The cortical potential was absent for 74 minutes, while the lumbar spinogram was always recordable.

Upon unclamping, the cortical response reappeared, with reduced amplitude, prolonged latency and abnormal morphology. On awakening, the patient presented with paraplegia and dissociated sensory loss below T 10–T 11. No sign of neurological improvement was apparent during the following three months, apart from the recovery from spinal shock. In the second unfavorable case, a man, the intraoperative scalp potential was lost 14 minutes after aortic clamping and was never recovered. The patient died.

Discussion

Analysis of the SEP changes in patients who had bad outcomes, compared with SEP changes in patients with favorable outcomes, suggests the following considerations.

Thirty minutes was the longest period of absent cortical SEP tolerated by patients without neurological complications. The disappearance of the cortical response did not immediately follow the aortic occlusion in most cases, and delays were as long as 25 minutes. Both spinal and peripheral nerve ischemia occurred. The lumbar potential was essential in distinguishing between the two.

Therefore it may be suggested that 30 minutes from the disappearance of the cortical potential is the maximal safe limit of aortic clamping, in the absence of distal perfusion adjuncts. The safe time allowed for operative occlusion of the aorta (30 to 55 minutes in our series) varies as a function of the time required for the cortical SEP to become undetectable. SEPs, therefore, appear to be a useful method of providing noninvasive spinal cord monitoring and able to give information of great relevance for the surgical management of these conditions.

It is commonly said that SEPs evoked by electrical stimulation of nerves in the lower limbs ascend the spinal cord mainly in the dorsal columns and in the dorsal spinocervical and spinocerebellar tracts and fail to test function of the entire cord. However, in acute situations of spinal cord ischemia, SEPs appear to be quite reliable indicators of global spinal cord function, even though in aortic cross-clamping the expected damage is more likely to occur in the anterior cord because of the sparseness and variability of segmental vessels feeding the anterior spinal artery[3].

References

1. Chiappa KH (Ed) (1983) Evoked potentials in clinical medicine. Raven Press Books Ltd, New York
2. Coles JC, Wilson GJ, Sima AF, Klement P, Tait GA, Williams WG, Baird RJ (1983) Intraoperative management of thoracic aortic aneurysm. J Thorac Cardiovasc Surg 85: 292–299
3. Grundy BL (1985) Intraoperative applications of evoked responses. In: Owen J, Davis H (eds) Evoked potential testing. Grune and Stratton Inc, Orlando, pp 159–212
4. Svensson LG, Rickards E, Coull A, Rogers G, Fimmel CJ, Hinder RA (1986) Relationship of spinal cord blood flow to vascular anatomy during thoracic aortic cross-clamping and shunting. J Thorac Cardiovasc Surg 91: 71–78
5. Szilagyi DE, Hageman JH, Smith RF, Elliott JP (1978) Spinal cord damage in surgery of the abdominal aorta. Surgery 83: 38–56

Subclavian Steal: Diagnostic Value of Reactive Hyperemia During Visual and Auditory Evoked Potential Recordings

M. G. SINATRA*, L. CARENINI**

* Fondazione don Gnocchi, Milano (Italy)
** Istituto Neurologico "C. Besta", Milano (Italy)

Introduction

Subclavian steal syndrome was described some decades ago by Contorni[4] and Reivich et al.[13] as a peculiar phenomenon due to a hemodynamic mechanism and characterized by reversal of blood flow through the vertebral artery. This particular condition is sometimes asymptomatic, and the only finding that make it suspect is different pulses in the two arms. Upper limb exercise can precipitate the steal and produce an increased pressure gradient between the pre-stenotic and post-stenotic portions of the vessel affected by the obstruction. Dynamic exercise or reactive hyperemia may therefore be useful as a provocative test for clinical evaluation[14] or in conjunction with directional Doppler sonography[11] and angiography[8].

Of the noninvasive examinations, directional Doppler sonography is quite reliable in detecting reversal of blood flow through the vertebral artery[17]; but there are few diagnostic tools that evaluate the effects of such a blood flow abnormality on brainstem structures.

Auditory brainstem responses (ABR), as a technique able to give objective information on brainstem structures crossed by auditory pathways, have been used to assess patients with brainstem strokes[15] and reversible ischemic attacks[9, 12]. The results mainly showed that ABR may be useful in the diagnostic and prognostic evaluation of brainstem ischemic events.

We have attempted to enhance the diagnostic sensitivity of evoked potentials by obtaining recordings in conjunction with a provocative test in two patients with asymptomatic subclavian steal in whom ABR were normal under standard conditions. In the same way, visual evoked potentials (VEP) were recorded in both patients in order to examine the brain structures supplied by terminal branches of the vertebral-basilar system.

Methods

ABR and VEP were recorded with Amplaid MK 7 equipment, in two sessions separated by an interval of a few days.

ABR method. Silver-silver chloride electrodes filled with electrolyte gel were applied to the vertex and mastoids; a midfrontal electrode served as ground. Electrode impedance was maintained below 3 KOhm. Alternating polarity clicks of 100 µs were presented monaurally through audiological TDH 39 earphones at the rate of 11/s and at the intensity of 70 dB s.l. without contralateral masking. EEG activity was recorded from the vertex and ipsilateral mastoid. Analysis time was 15 ms. The responses were filtered with a bandpass of 0.2 to 3.0 KHz. Two recordings of 2,000 averaged responses were obtained from each ear. The input sensitivity was maintained below 20 µV. During recordings patients were in the supine position.

VEP method. Platinum needle electrodes were placed on the scalp according to the Queen Square system[2]. Impedance was maintained below 3 KOhm. Recordings were taken in a darkened room, where patients were seated on a chair and instructed to fix their eyes on a red dot at the center of the screen. Each eye was tested separately by full-field stimulation, recording from MO (midfrontal-occipital), and left and right occipital (LO-RO). A black-and-white checkerboard pattern-reversal stimulation was carried out at a frequency of 1.6 Hz with a stimulating field of 12°31' of the visual angle. Each square subtended 55.02 min of arc. Contrast was 100%. The VEP signal was amplified with 1 to 200 Hz bandpass. Analysis time was 250 ms. One hundred responses were averaged for each set.

Three sets of evoked responses (ABR and VEP) were obtained for each patient, before, during and about 20 min after the provocative test. Reactive hyperemia was used to prevent artifacts due to dynamic exercises of the upper limb. A blood pressure cuff was applied to the arm ipsilateral to the subclavian artery stenosis, inflated to 200 mmHg for about 10 min, and soon after deflated at the same time as began recording, ABR and VEP obtained during reactive hyperemia were compared with those obtained before and after the provocative test.

Case 1. A right-handed, 49-year-old man had, 10 days before admission, experienced a left hemiparesis with almost full recovery within 24 h. Two days after the hemiparesis a CT scan showed a right frontal-parietal hypodense lesion. Upon admission, neurological examination showed a slight hemiparesis of the left side involving the face and limbs with hyperreflexia. No sign or symptom due to brainstem dysfunction was found. Neuropsychological evaluation showed only some impairment in Rey's figure copying test. Blood pressure values in the two arms were repeatedly different (150/100 for the right and 130/100 for the left). As Doppler sonography had previously shown, digital intravenous arteriography demonstrated bilateral stenosis of the internal carotid arteries (severe on the right and slight on the left). Furthermore, a left subclavian steal with reversal of blood flow through the left vertebral artery was noted. At the time of admission the patient had been receiving anticoagulant therapy for a week. Hearing level and visual acuity were normal.

Case 2. A right-handed, 52-year-old man had, 2 months before admission, complained of speech disturbances and slight motor impairment of the right limbs with full recovery within 2 h. He had never complained of any symptom referable to brainstem dysfunction. The neurological examination was normal. Pressure values differed greatly between the two arms (100/70 on the right and 150/100 on the left). CT scan was normal even after injection of contrast medium. Doppler sonography showed occlusion of the subclavian artery with reversal of blood flow through the vertebral artery on the right side. Angiography confirmed this finding and in addition demonstrated some irregularity of the intima at the bifurcation of the internal carotid on the left and at the top of the basilar artery. At the time of admission the patient had been receiving antiplatelet treatment for 2 months. Audiological testing showed only a slight impairment in both ears. Visual acuity was normal.

Results

In both patients the ABR recordings failed to show any abnormality under standard conditions: all waves were well recognizable and interpeak latencies were within normal values. During the provocative test a completely different pattern was seen: all but the first waves disappeared or decreased in amplitude. Similar findings were obtained from both ears in each patient, but with more serious abnormalities in case 1. About 20 min after reactive hyperemia, two more sets of ABR were recorded for both patients, and the same findings and interpeak latencies were observed as under standard conditions (Figs. 1 and 2).

To verify whether ABR abnormalities found during reactive hyperemia were due to phenomena other than hemodynamic events, ABR recordings were repeated after carrying out the provocative test on the arm contralateral to the side of the subclavian artery stenosis. No abnormality was found either during or after the test. Throughout the recording session neither patient reported any symptoms referable to brainstem dysfunction, even when ABR abnormalities appeared on the screen. Both patients complained of slight discomfort in the arm compressed by the sphygmomanometer cuff.

No modification in VEP occurred during reactive hyperemia in either patient. An asymmetry in amplitude of P 100, which was lower on the left, was found in lateral-occipital areas in all the recordings obtained for case 1.

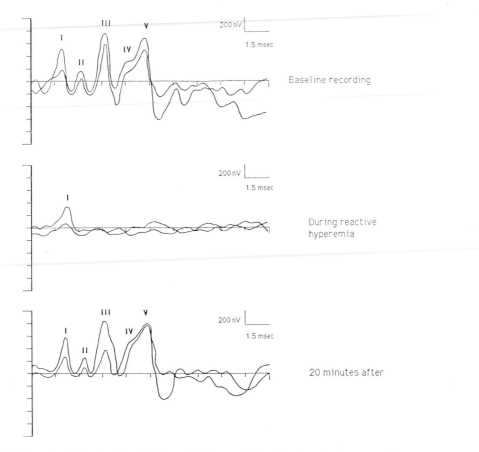

Fig. 1. Case 1. ABR obtained before, during and 20 min after the provocative test
performed on the same side as the subclavian artery stenosis

Discussion

The occurrence of ABR abnormalities during the provocative test in our
two patients with asymptomatic subclavian steal shows that hemodynamic
mechanisms can modify the progression of impulses through the auditory
pathways of the brainstem. The role of hemodynamic events in producing
such abnormalities is confirmed by the lack of ABR modifications when
the same test was performed on the arm contralateral to the subclavian
stenosis. ABRs recorded about 20 min after the provocative test were normal in both patients, which showed that impairment of the brainstem structures due to a decreased blood flow was transient and completely reversible.

It may be hypothesized that under standard conditions, reversal of blood
flow through the vertebral artery, as documented by angiography, does
not produce inadequate blood supply to the brainstem. The provocative

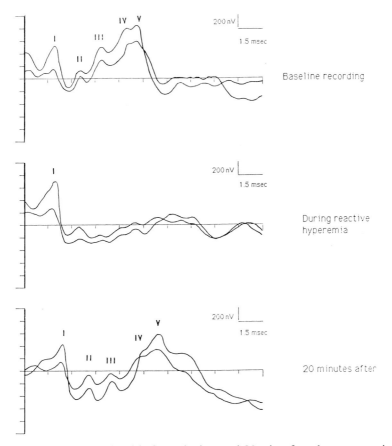

Fig. 2. Case 2. ABR obtained before, during and 20 min after the provocative test
performed on the same side as the subclavian artery stenosis

test, however, gives rise to a critical drop in blood flow and causes functional
suppression but not irreversible damage to nerve cells. In our two subjects
the main expression of this functional damage was the disappearance or
flattening of most components of auditory evoked responses. The initial
response of nerve cells is probably a suppression of the electrical activity
that we can detect in electrophysiologic recordings.

During the recording sessions, neither patient complained of any symptom referable to brainstem dysfunction.

In theory, recording of ABR with patients in the supine position could
have limited the drop in blood flow to the brainstem and accounted for
the absence of symptoms. However, this hypothesis was not confirmed by
VEP recordings; although visual responses were obtained in a sitting position, no clinical event occurred.

The specific ABR abnormalities found during reactive hyperemia consisted of disappearance or flattening of all waves but the first one. As described by Duvernoy[5], the brainstem structures crossed by auditory pathways are supplied by branches of basilar, vertebral and posterior inferior cerebellar arteries. Our findings show that good perfusion of the hypothesized generators of ABR waves is necessary to obtain clearly recognizable peaks. Unfortunately, our results do not help to settle the debate as to whether the second wave is generated by the brainstem[3, 6, 7, 10]; both the hypothesized generators of this wave, the 8th cranial nerve and cochlear nucleus, can be perfused via the same branches of the basilar artery. The 8th nerve is perfused by the anterior inferior cerebellar artery and the internal auditory artery; the cochlear nucleus is supplied by the anterior inferior cerebellar artery. The question is further complicated by the fact that little is known about how many and which vessels are involved in the subclavian steal. Visual evoked responses were not modified by the provocative test in either patient. This finding could be due either to a lower sensitivity of VEP in detecting a transient ischemic impairment of the brain parenchyma or to the fact that the visual areas supplied by the posterior cerebral arteries were not involved in the steal. The asymmetry in amplitude of P 100 found in all recordings for case 1 can be explained by the ischemic lesion demonstrated by CT scan[1, 16].

In conclusion, our findings suggest that the use of the provocative test during ABR recordings can be useful to detect subclinical and transient ischemic impairment of brainstem function and to document the role of the subclavian steal in producing such effects.

References

1. Barret G, Blumhardt LD, Halliday AM, Halliday E, Kriss A (1976) A paradox in the lateralization of the visual evoked response. Nature 261: 253–255
2. Chatrian GE (1984) American electroencephalographic society guidelines for clinical evoked potentials studies. J Clin Neurophysiol 1: 3–53
3. Chiappa KH (ed) Evoked potentials in clinical medicine. Raven Press, New York, pp 145–156
4. Contorni L (1960) Il circolo collaterale vertebrobasilare nella obliterazione della arteria succlavia alle sue origini. Min Chir 15: 268–275
5. Duvernoy HM (1978) Human brainstem vessels. Springer, Berlin Heidelberg New York
6. Garg BP, Markand ON, Bustion PF (1982) Brainstem auditory evoked responses in hereditary motor-sensory neuropathy: site of origin of wave II. Neurology 32: 1017–1019
7. Lacey DJ, Terplan K (1984) Correlating auditory evoked and brainstem histologic abnormalities in infantile Gaucher's disease. Neurology (Cleveland) 34: 539–541
8. Marshall RJ, Mantini EL (1965) Dynamics of the collateral circulation in patients with subclavian steal. Circulation 36: 249–254

9. Maurer K, Marneros A, Schäfer E, Leitner H (1969) Early auditory evoked potentials, (EAEP) in vertebral basilar insufficiency. Arch Psychiatr Nervenkr 227

10. Moller AR, Jannetta B, Bennett M, Moller MB (1981) Intracranially recorded responses from the human auditory nerve: new insights into the origin of brainstem evoked potentials (BSEPs). Electroencephalogr Clin Neurophysiol 52: 18–27

11. Mozersky DJ, Branes RW, Summer DS, Strandness DE (1973) Hemodynamics of innominate artery occlusion. Ann Surg 178: 123–127

12. Ragazzoni A, Amantini A, Rossi L, Pagnini P, Arnetoli G, Marini P, Nencioni C, Versari A, Zappoli R (1982) Brainstem auditory evoked potentials and vertebral-basilar reversible ischemic attacks. In: Courjon J, Mauguiere F, Ravol M (eds) Clinical applications of evoked potentials in neurology. Raven Press, New York, pp 187–194

13. Reivich M, Holling E, Roberts B, Toole JF (1961) Reversal of blood flow through the vertebral artery and its effect on cerebral circulation. N Engl J Med 265: 878–885

14. Sharon M, Asinger RW, Hodges M (1981) Reactive hyperemia for the clinical diagnosis of subclavian steal syndrome: report of a case. Stroke 12: 369–371

15. Stern BJ, Drumholz A, Weiss HD, Goldstein P, Harris KC (1982) Evaluation of brainstem stroke using brainstem auditory evoked responses. Stroke 13: 705–711

16. Streletz LJ, Base SH, Roeshman RM, Schatz NJ, Savino PJ (1981) Visual evoked potentials in occipital lobe lesions. Arch Neurol 38: 80–85

17. Von Reutern GM, Büdingen HJ, Freund HJ (1976) Dopplersonographische Diagnostik von Stenosen und Verschlüssen der Vertebral-Arterien und des Subclavian-Steal Syndroms. Arch Psychiatr Nervenkr 222: 209–222

Utility and Uncertainties of Evoked Potential Monitoring in the Intensive Care Unit

F. Mauguière*, L. Garcia Larrea*, O. Bertrand**

* EEG Department, Hôpital Neurologique, Lyon (France),
** INSERM Unité 280, Lyon (France)

Patients admitted to a neurological intensive care unit (ICU) often undergo sudden variations of their homeostasis which may lead to important changes in their clinical status and probability of survival. Up to now most studies aimed at evaluating the prognostic significance of single or daily recordings of early somatosensory (SEPs) or brainstem auditory (BAEPs) evoked potentials in coma. Electrophysiological assessment of comatose patients with EP techniques is peculiarly needed in head-injured patients receiving continuous infusions of short-acting barbiturates which modify brainstem reflexes and EEG activity with little or no effect on early SEPs or BAEPs[14, 20, 31, 32, 42, 45, 46]. A finding common to most of these investigations was that outcome is invariably poor in comatose patients with abnormal BAEP waves or bilateral absence of the contralateral parietal N 20 evoked by median nerve stimulation[6, 9, 17, 18, 27, 29, 36, 38, 39, 47, 51]. However, several investigators have pointed out that in many cases the information provided by a single EP recording might not be of prognostic significance in the ICU setting, especially when responses are normal[1, 9, 11, 39]. This statement is illustrated by our SEP data from a series of 53 comatose patients (Glasgow score < 7) as shown in Table 1. This table shows that a poor outcome is to be expected when the contralateral N 20 component of the SEP is absent bilaterally after stimulation of the median nerve; but it also demonstrates that a poor outcome may occur in patients with normal N 20 on both sides.

Two factors may explain the poor prognostic value of a single, or even daily, EP recording. First, a sudden change in the patient's homeostasis such as an increase of intracranial pressure (ICP) may cause death only a few minutes after normal EPs were recorded. Second, a slow but steady degradation of EPs with a timecourse of several hours may be unnoticed if the recording session takes place when latencies and amplitudes, though

Table 1. *Outcome (One-month Follow-up)*

Parietal N 20		Good recovery	Moderate disability	Severe disability	Vegetative state	Death
Absent (both sides)	21	0	0	3	4	14
Present (both sides)	32	4	5	12	5	6
Total	53	4	5	15	9	20

progressively degrading, still remain within normal limits. Thus there is a need for EP monitoring systems designed for rapidly repeated EP recordings at the patient's bed-side. Moreover, data provided by such systems must be immediately available and reliable enough to support therapeutic decisions. As stated by Hacke (1985)[19]: "single examination, or repeated examinations at long intervals, or storing of continuously obtained data for later interpretation should not be regarded as monitoring".

A System for High-Rate Sequential BAEP Recording and Feature Extraction

Several systems for automatic recordings of EPs have been proposed[5, 30, 33, 37]. In this chapter we report our experience with a system designed by one of us (Bertrand) which permits continuous monitoring of BAEPs. One of the reasons we chose to focus our research first on BAEPs is that homeostatic variations which occur in deeply comatose head-injured patients have in common their ability to damage the brainstem. The utility of BAEPs in functional assessment of the brainstem has been emphasized in various conditions, including coma and brain death[6, 21, 28, 41, 45, 48], provided that direct peripheral damage to the auditory transduction apparatus or VIIIth nerve has been ruled out. Moreover, since their first description in humans[24], BAEPs proved to be fairly reliable in detecting and localizing brainstem lesions[11, 15, 16, 22, 43, 44, 47].

This system consists of a one-channel EP device coupled to a microcomputer which controls all operations (see[3], for a detailed description). The recording procedure is a standard one. Electrodes are either Ag/AgCl disks fixed with collodion or sterilized subdermal needles. They are placed at CZ (connected with the positive input of the preamplifier) and over the mastoid process ipsilateral to the stimulated ear (negative input). A third electrode over the contralateral mastoid process serves as ground. The stimuli, delivered through an ear-inserted transducer, are non-filtered alternating clicks of 80 or 90 dB HL, generated by square wave electrical pulses of 100 µsec duration at a rate of 20/sec. BAEPs are obtained over an analysis time of 12.8 msec (bin width 50 µsec) and filtered by the analog filters of the EP device with a bandpass of 150–1,300 Hz (-3 dB cutoff, slope of 6 dB per octave). Evoked potential averaging is performed by blocks of 200 single trials, with automatic artifact rejection. The number of repetitions for each averaged BAEP is thus a multiple of 200. The time interval between two successive BAEPs is selected on the computer. Raw data are transferred to the computer, sequentially displayed on a color video-screen, processed, and stored on a floppy disk.

An optimal digital filter, based on Wiener filtering theory[13, 49, 50], is calculated by the computer for each BAEP and reactualized after every averaging session. The adaptive Wiener filter (AWF) is computed from an ensemble of N successive BAEPs and applied to the very last BAEP. Then a new averaged BAEP is acquired, the AWF is updated from the N last BAEP and applied to the very last one. For routine recordings in the ICU, AWF is usually estimated from a sequence of N = 5 successive BAEPs. Interpretable traces can be obtained after 200 to 400 stimuli, thus reducing recording time to 10–20 sec for each individual BAEP. The time interval between recording sessions is usually two minutes but can be modified at any moment during monitoring. Fig. 1 illustrates the effect of AWF on a sequence of BAEPs contaminated by intermittent low-frequency noise.

Our main concern in monitoring BAEPs was to follow on-line latency changes of waves I, III, and V. Therefore an algorithm was developed to automatically track these positive peaks. At the beginning of the monitoring session several standard BAEPs are recorded to check that responses are reproducible. BAEPs are first studied separately for each ear, and the side with the better responses is selected for subsequent monitoring. Waves I, III, and V are identified by the examiner and their latencies measured by using a cursor. Latency values are stored and serve as references for automatic peak detection. After these preliminary maneuvers sequential BAEPs are obtained in an automatic mode at the chosen rate. "Trend curves" of peak latencies as well as the last twenty individual BAEPs are continuously displayed on the computer screen at the patient's bedside. It is also possible to automatically measure wave amplitude (from peak to following trough) and to have the results displayed on the screen.

Several analog physiological signals such as intracranial pressure (ICP), mean (MAP) or systolic (SAP) arterial blood pressure and body temperature can also be digitized and averaged over the stimulation period required to obtain each BAEP. These values are then stored and plotted on the computer screen in synchrony with BAEP latencies.

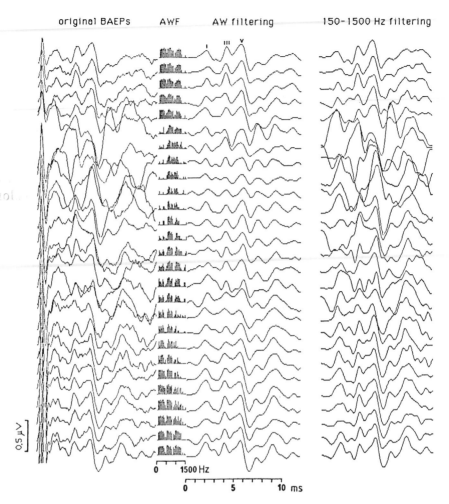

Fig. 1. Effects of Adaptative Wiener Filtering on a sequence of BAEPs contaminated by transient low-frequency noise (muscle activity). Original BAEPs (left column) are recorded every two minutes after 200 stimulations. Responses are transiently blurred (from trace 6 to trace 12) by low-frequency muscle activity. During this period of time the transfer function of the Adaptive Wiener Filter (AWF) eliminates the low frequency noise between 0 and 400 Hertz. In spite of a non-negligible effect of AWF upon the amplitude of the response, peaks I, III, and V can be accurately detected and tracked during this period

BAEP Deterioration Does Not Necessarily Mean that Brainstem Is Suffering

The first challenge of EP monitoring is to differentiate response changes which are clinically important and should be rapidly identified to improve patient care from those which are falsely alarming. Our experience with

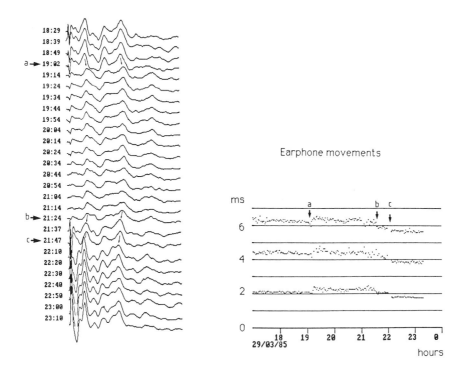

Fig. 2. Latency shifts of BAEPs due to earphone movements. In (a) the earphone was pulled out of the external auditory meatus and then pushed into it (b) and (c). The plotting of wave I, III, and V (right) clearly shows that I–V interpeak delay remains constant in spite of latency shift and amplitude decrease of all components related to the change of stimulation level. Serial BAEPs displayed on the left side of the figure were obtained after 200 stimulations and selected every ten minutes for illustration

the above described BAEP monitoring system now includes 40 comatose patients, mostly head-injured (76%), with a mean number of 1030 BAEPs per patient. A clear conclusion is that BAEP changes related to technical factors, shifts of body temperature and direct action of drugs upon the nervous system are frequently encountered in such patients. This is so partly because our series includes deeply comatose and highly medicated patients, but these are the patients who most need EP monitoring. On admission to the ICU all our patients had a Glasgow Coma Score less than seven. When barbiturate anesthesia was used to control ICP, patients' thiopental blood levels were usually maintained between 15 and 25 mg/l. Some patients were under an anesthetic combination of lidocaine and thiopental, with lidocaine blood levels between 10 and 25 mg/l[2]. In addition, occasional intravenous doses of mannitol, thiopental or gamma-hydroxy butyrate were used to control acute episodes of high ICP when necessary.

Some of the BAEP changes not directly related to brainstem deterioration are easy to identify. For instance, changes of stimulation level due to earphone movements cause rapid latency shifts of all waves without change of the I–V interpeak latency. This problem can be immediately corrected by checking earphone position (see Fig. 2). Conductive hearing loss related to endotracheal intubation did not present a real problem in our patients, probably because all of them were under chronic ventilatory assistance when BAEP monitoring was carried out. On the contrary, two factors, body temperature and sedative drugs, caused BAEP changes mimicking those observed during brainstem deterioration; their effects will be described successively.

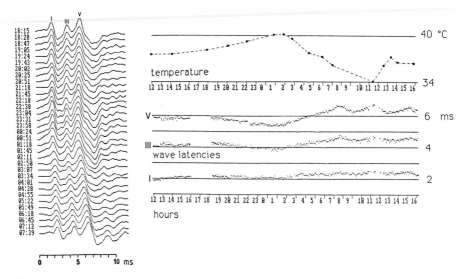

Fig. 3. Latency changes related to temperature variations during coma. This figure illustrates the effects on BAEP latencies of hyperthermia up to 40 °C (from 18:00–01:00 hours) and of temperature decrease from hyper- to hypothermia down to 34 °C (01:00–11:00 h). Traces displayed on the left of the figure were recorded after 200 stimulations and filtered with AWF; they were selected in the sequence obtained between 18:15 h and 7:39 h. The plotting of trend curves of peaks I, III, and V latencies (right) shows that fluctuations of BAEP latencies closely parallel those of body temperature. Note that between 07:00 h and 11:00 h there was a decrease of BAEP latencies suggesting that during this period body temperature transiently increased. Since no temperature data were available during this period this interpretation remains conjectural. This example emphasizes the statement that EP monitoring requires concomitant monitoring of all the biological parameters that may influence the responses. The effect of temperature on waves I, III, and V is cumulative, the overall I–V interval latency change being 0.16 msec/°C

Body Temperature

Fig. 3 illustrates the finding that temperature shifts can be responsible for BAEP changes very similar to those seen under pathological conditions. Long-lasting changes in the latencies of waves I, III, and V related to a fall in body temperature can be confused with deterioration of brainstem function due to inadequate cerebral perfusion pressure (CPP) (vide infra). The highest and lowest temperatures recorded in our patients were 40 and 34 °C. Between these two values BAEP changes in relation to temperature variations are very stereotyped, with a progressive increase of all wave latencies as temperature decreases. This effect is cumulative from peripheral to central components: wave I only shows a 0.05 msec/°C mean latency shift, while waves III and V exhibit variations of 0.14 and 0.21 msec/°C respectively, thus giving a mean shift of 0.16 ms/°C for the I–V interval. This increase of BAEP latencies is reversible when body temperature rises. Thus, temperature monitoring is essential to avoid misleading interpretations of BAEP changes during continuous monitoring.

Drugs

In our series of seven patients under continuous infusion of thiopental in monotherapy, it was found that this procedure does not cause BAEP latency shifts when barbiturate serum levels are in the usual therapeutic range (see above). Similarly, no BAEP changes are detected after bolus i.v. injections of thiopental up to 5 mg/kg of body weight, but the drug's blood levels are not systematically controlled in this condition. On the contrary, consistent BAEP latency shifts similar to those of preterminal brainstem deterioration can be produced by a combination of lidocaine and thiopental. Figure 4 illustrates a peculiarly dramatic BAEP deterioration probably facilitated by transient thiopental overdose with this drug combination. In ten patients we observed similar changes of various degrees at thiopental blood levels that do not cause any BAEP change when this drug is used alone. The increase of BAEP latencies is related to lidocaine dosage and is cumulative, with an increase of I–V interpeak latency up to 2 msec. Most of the studies regarding the effect of drugs on EPs have been done with single agents[4, 14, 23, 46]; our finding indicates that caution must be exercised in extrapolating these results to patients treated with combinations of drugs.

Time Course and Pathophysiology of BAEP Changes During Brainstem Deterioration in Coma

Data were collected in eight head-injured patients whose BAEPs, ICP, and MAP were continuously monitored until brain death. None of them presented preterminal temperature modifications that per se could have in-

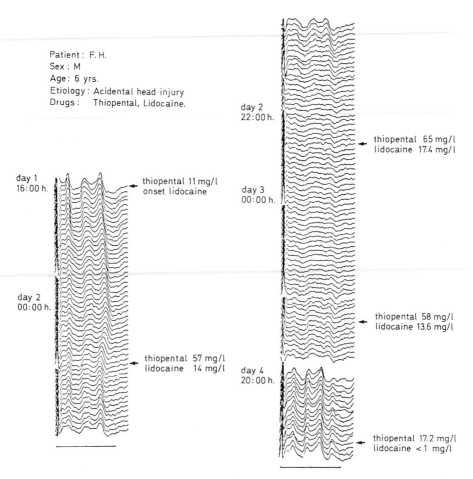

Patient : F.H.
Sex : M
Age: 6 yrs.
Etiology : Acidental head injury
Drugs :   Thiopental, Lidocaine.

day 2
22:00 h.

← thiopental 65 mg/l
  lidocaine 17.4 mg/l

day 1
16:00 h.

← thiopental 11 mg/l
  onset lidocaine

day 3
00:00 h.

day 2
00:00 h.

← thiopental 58 mg/l
  lidocaine 13.6 mg/l

← thiopental 57 mg/l
  lidocaine 14 mg/l

day 4
20:00 h.

← thiopental 17.2 mg/l
  lidocaine < 1 mg/l

Fig. 4. BAEP changes with high doses of thiopental and lidocaine. In this patient increasing blood levels of lidocaine and sodium thiopental, administered in continuous intravenous infusion, are associated with a progressive deterioration of BAEPs manifested by latency increase and amplitude fall of all components. BAEPs are almost abolished at 65 mg/l of thiopental and 17.4 mg/l of lidocaine. Drug interruption on day 4 is followed by complete recovery of normal BAEP waveforms. Final outcome was good. Note that nearly the same drug blood levels correspond to very different aspects of BAEPs in the right and left columns. This suggests that, because of drug kinetics, identical blood levels of sedative drugs can have different functional effects that are probably related to different concentrations in the brain

fluenced BAEP evolution. In all of them thiopental and lidocaine blood levels were monitored. Two different patterns of BAEP deterioration with different pathophysiological significance can be described.

Simultaneous Deterioration of Waves I, III, and V

This pattern was observed in five patients. BAEP changes occurred either gradually over several hours or suddenly in a few minutes. The disappearance of BAEP waves was preceded by a progressive delay of waves I, III, and V peak latencies in two cases. In one of these patients wave I persisted for five hours after complete abolition of wave V. Wave V disappeared when CPP was 15 mmHg, while wave I could be identified with a progressive increase in its peak latency until CPP was 8 mmHg. In three patients with sudden BAEP deterioration, all waves disappeared simultaneously without previous latency shifts.

In such patients low cerebral perfusion pressure (< 40 mmHg), due either to a fall of MAP or to combined increase of ICP and decrease of MAP, was constantly observed when BAEPs definitely disappeared. The time courses of CPP decrease and BAEP changes were closely correlated. In the two patients with progressive increases in latencies of waves I, III, and V, there was a slow and steady reduction of mean CPP values. The duration of BAEP degradation was of 10 and 18 hrs, respectively, and its onset was associated with a fall in CPP. In both cases I-V interpeak latencies were normal before hemodynamic deterioration. Conversely, in the three patients with sudden disappearance of the BAEPs, CPP fell to dangerously low values in a short period of time (10, 30, and 50 minutes, respectively).

Simultaneous deterioration of waves I, III, and V is consistent with ongoing ischemia affecting both the brainstem and the cochlear nerve or cochlea. All these structures are supplied by the vertebrobasilar circulation[7] and are likely to be simultaneously affected by a CPP decrease in this vascular territory. Although vascular autoregulation keeps cerebral blood flow (CBF) roughly constant in the presence of CPP values between 40 and 150 mmHg, vascular autoregulatory mechanisms can be impaired in patients with severe head injuries. Recording neuronal activity with BAEPs is a useful adjunct to the indirect assessment of CBF provided by CPP monitoring.

Sohmer et al.[40] observed in cats that wave I could still be present after all brainstem components of the BAEP had disappeared during slow controlled decrease of CPP. Our data also suggest that, in spite of simultaneous deterioration, different BAEP waves are not affected to the same degree during progressive ischemia. Brainstem components of the response are more sensitive than wave I. This statement does not hold in case of a sudden fall of CPP, as for example in the case of cardiac arrest. In such conditions total abolition of BAEPs may be due to early, and possibly selective, anoxic necrosis of the cochlea. Indeed, total autolysis of the organ of Corti has been reported in a brain dead patient whose BAEPs were absent[26]. Isolated ischemic damage to peripheral receptors was also proposed by Brunko

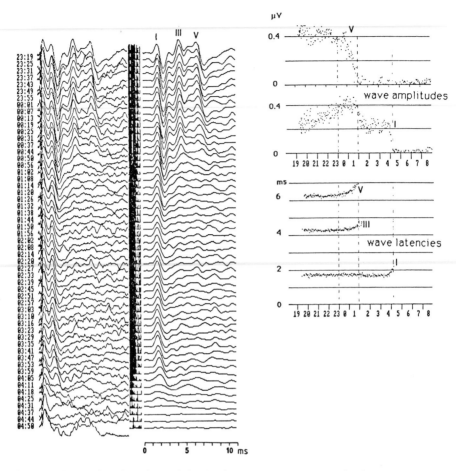

Fig. 5. Isolated deterioration of the brainstem components of BAEPs (Waves III to V) in brain death. In this case of brain death related to an episode of intracranial hypertension, wave V is the first to be affected and cannot be visually identified after 00:37 hours on original (left column) or AWF filtered traces (right column) obtained after 200 stimulations. Automatic tracking of wave V amplitude and latency (right) is not possible after 01:00 h but abnormal evolution of this peak with latency increase and amplitude decrease is detectable on trend curves plotted at 24:00 h. Our preliminary experience suggests that in comatose patients at risk for acute intracranial hypertension due to brain edema or a supratentorial space-occupying lesion, this selective deterioration of wave V is alarming and indicates upper brainstem injury due to increasing intracranial pressure. The second event of BAEP degradation is represented by a latency increase followed by complete disappearance of wave III. Wave I, reflecting activity of the VIIIth nerve, persists until 04:00 h. Note that automatic measurement of wave I amplitude demonstrates that this component begins to increase before any detectable change of wave V

et al.[8] to explain the absence of BAEPs after cardiac arrest despite normal early SEPs and anatomically normal brainstem and thalamus on neuro-pathological examination.

Deterioration of Waves III and V with Preserved Wave I

In this pattern, BAEP changes were initially limited to the brainstem components while wave I was preserved in 3 patients (Fig. 5). None of them had very low CPP values when components III and V disappeared. In all, wave I persisted for several hours after the loss of all other components and disappeared either when MAP fell to values less than 50 mmHg or when ICP became higher than 80 mmHg. Before terminal BAEP changes the I–V interpeak latencies were within normal limits. The changes in waves III and V could not be related to any consistent modification of the CPP. These 3 patients also presented a peculiar BAEP pattern with an increase in wave I amplitude concurrent with the progressive latency increase and amplitude decrease of wave V (Fig. 5). This feature was not encountered, even transiently, in any other patients in our series.

In post-traumatic coma, sequential disappearance of BAEPs from wave V to wave I suggests progressive rostro-caudal deterioration of brainstem function related to elevated ICP[34, 35]. However, on the basis of ICP monitoring, isolated intracranial hypertension was manifest as a probable cause of brain death in only one of our three cases. Of the other two patients, one showed only a minimal ICP increase which coincided with a notable decrease in arterial pressure (AP). In the other patients no variations of ICP or AP were recorded even though BAEP provided unequivocal evidence of brainstem deterioration with preserved wave I. At autopsy, the first of these two patients had bilateral transtentorial herniation of the temporal lobes. Divergences between BAEP and ICP findings have also been reported by Hall *et al.*[21] in a comatose patient whose BAEPs were preserved despite elevated ICP, a situation that was not uncommon in our series. This supports the view that extradural monitoring of supratentorial ICP is less reliable than BAEP monitoring to assess brainstem injury during coma.

Isolated preservation of wave I has been previously reported in brain death[18, 27, 41]. Increase of wave I amplitude concomitant to deterioration of all brainstem components has also been reported in isolated records by Starr[41] and Hall *et al.*[21]. Explanatory hypotheses include acoustic reflex inhibition due to a brainstem lesion, already discussed and discarded by Hall[20]; post-ischemic enhancement of the auditory nerve compound action potential[25]; and interruption of inhibitory centrifugal pathways such as the olivo-cochlear bundle[12, 21]. Our data provide complementary information concerning the time course of wave I preterminal changes by showing that amplitude increase can begin before any electrophysiological evidence of brainstem dysfunction (Fig. 5).

Concluding Remarks

With the present state of the art, three conclusions can be drawn from our experience. First, signal acquisition and data processing can now be reliably performed at the patient's bedside in order to obtain rapid sequential BAEP recordings. Second, continuous monitoring represents the only means of detecting significant trends in BAEP evolution which are not necessarily associated with definitely abnormal individual responses. Third, evolving BAEP patterns due to brainstem deterioration as well as falsely alarming changes related to drug and temperature shifts can be identified. The question of whether BAEP monitoring could improve final outcomes of head-injured patients deserves further investigation. Ethical considerations preclude the possibility or performing such an evaluation by comparing outcomes in a randomized series of patients with or without monitoring. Our routine experience is that members of the ICU medical staff now use the information provided by BAEPs to promptly correct the deviations from homeostasis responsible for BAEP changes. An obvious next step is to continuously monitor EP components like the SEP N 20 that are generated at levels above the brainstem and therefore seem likely to be affected earlier than BAEPs when a patient's condition is deteriorating.

References

1. Anderson DC, Scott B, Rockswold GL (1984) Multimodality evoked potentials in closed head trauma. Arch Neurol 41: 369–374
2. Artru F, Jourdan C, Ferry M, Montarry M, Roche P, Deleuze R (1986) Protection cérébrale par perfusion continue de lidocaïne. In: Les Comas (Soc de réanimation de Langue Française Bruxelles, May 29th–31st), pp 75–79
3. Bertrand O, Garcia Larrea L, Artru F, Mauguière F, Pernier J (1987) Brainstem monitoring: a system for high rate BAEP sequential monitoring and feature extraction. Electroencephalogr Clin Neurophysiol 68: 433–445
4. Bobbin RP, May JG, Lemoine RL (1979) Effects of pentobarbital and ketamine on brain-stem auditory potentials. Arch Otolaryngol 105: 467–470
5. Boston JR, Deneault LG (1984) Sensory evoked potentials: a system for clinical testing and patient monitoring. Int J Clin Monitoring and Computing 1: 13–19
6. Brewer CC, Resnick DM (1984) The value of BAEPs in assessment of the comatose patient. In: Nodar RH, Barber C (eds) Evoked potentials II. Butterworths Publishers, Boston, pp 578–581
7. Brodal A (1969) Neurological anatomy. Oxford University Press, New York London Toronto

8. Brunko E, Delecluse F, Herbaut AG, Levivier M, Zegers de Beyl D (1985) Unusual pattern of somatosensory and brain-stem auditory evoked potentials after cardio-respiratory arrest. Electroencephalogr Clin Neurophysiol 62: 338–342

9. Cant BR, Hume AL, Judson JA, Shaw NA (1986) The assessment of severe head injury by short latency somatosensory and brain-stem auditory evoked potentials. Electroencephalogr Clin Neurophysiol 65: 188–195

10. Chiappa KH (1982) Brainstem auditory evoked potentials in clinical neurology. In: Courjon J, Mauguière F, Revol F (eds) Clinical applications of evoked potentials in neurology. Raven Press, New York, pp 169–175

11. Chiappa KH (1983) Brainstem auditory evoked potentials. Interpretation. In: Evoked potentials in clinical medicine. Raven Press, New York, pp 145–189

12. Desmedt JE (1962) Auditory evoked potentials from cochlea to cortex as interferenced by activation of the efferent olivo-cochlear bundle. J Acoust Soc Am 1478–1496

13. Doyle DJ (1975) Some comments on the use of Wiener filtering for the estimation of evoked potentials. Electroencephalogr Clin Neurophysiol 38: 533–534

14. Drummond JC, Todd MM, U HS (1985) The effect of high dose sodium thiopental on brain stem auditory and median nerve somatosensory evoked responses in humans. Anesthesiology 63: 249–254

15. Fischer C, Blanc A, Mauguière F, Courjon J (1981) Apport des potentiels évoqués auditifs précoces au diagnostic neurologique. Rev Neurol 137: 229–240

16. Fisher C, Mauguière F, Echallier JF, Tommasi M, Courjon J (1982) Brainstem acoustic evoked potentials in vascular and tumoral lesions of the brainstem. In: Courjon J, Mauguière F, Revol F (eds) Clinical applications of evoked potentials in neurology. Raven Press, New York, 32, pp 177–186

17. Facco E, Martini A, Zuccarello M, Agnoletto M, Giron GP (1985) Is the Auditory Brainstem Response (ABR) effective in the assessment coma? Electroencephalogr Clin Neurophysiol 62: 332–337

18. Goldie WD, Chiappa KH, Young RR, Brooks EB (1981) Brainstem auditory and short-latency somatosensory evoked responses in brain death. Neurology 31: 248–256

19. Hacke W (1985) Neuromonitoring. J Neurol 232: 125–133

20. Hall JW (1985) The effects of high-dose barbiturates on the acoustic reflex and auditory evoked responses. Acta Otolaryngol 100: 387–398

21. Hall JW, Mackey-Hargadine JR, Kim EE (1985) Auditory brainstem responses in determination of brain death. Arch Otolaryngol 111: 613–620

22. House JW, Brackmann DE (1979) Brainstem audiometry in neurotologic diagnosis. Arch Otolaryngol 105: 305–309

23. Javel E, Mouney DF, McGee JA, Walsh EJ (1982) Auditory brainstem responses during systemic infusion of lidocaine. Arch Otolaryngol 108: 71–76

24. Jewett DL, Romano MA, Williston JS (1970) Human auditory evoked potentials. Possible brainstem components detected on the scalp. Science 167: 1517–1518

25. Jones TA, Weidner WJ (1986) Effects of temperature and elevated intracranial pressure on peripheral and brainstem auditory responses in dogs. Exp Neurol 92: 1–12

26. Kaga K, Takamori A, Mizutani T, Nagai T, Marsh RR (1985) The auditory pathology of brain death as revealed by auditory evoked potentials. Ann Neurol 18: 360–364

27. Kallwellis G, Roder H, Rabending G (1980) Auditory evoked brainstem potentials in patients in coma and brain death. Electroencephalogr Clin Neurophysiol 50: 100 P

28. Karnaze DS, Weiner JM, Marshall LF (1985) Auditory evoked potentials in coma after closed head injury. A clinical-neurophysiological coma scale for predicting outcome. Neurology 35: 1122–1126

29. Lindsay KW, Carlin J, Kennedy I, Fry J, McInnes A, Teasdale GM (1981) Evoked potentials in severe head injury. Analysis and relation to outcome. J Neurol Neurosurg Psychiatry 44: 796–802

30. Maresch H, Pfurtscheller G (1983) Simultaneous measurement of auditory brainstem potentials and EEG spectra. Electroencephalogr Clin Neurophysiol 56: 531–533

31. Mauguière F (1982) Brainstem auditory and short-latency somatosensory evoked responses in coma and brain death. In: Touraine JL, Traeger J (eds) Transplantation and clinical immunology. Excerpta Medica, Amsterdam, 14, pp 238–250

32. Mauguière F, Grand C, Fischer C, Courjon J (1982) Aspects des potentiels évoqués auditifs et somésthésiques précoces dans les comas neurologiques et la mort cérébrale. Rev EEG Neurophysiol 12: 280–286

33. Maynard DE, Jenkinson JL (1984) The cerebral function analyzing monitor. Anesthesia 39: 678–690

34. Nagao S, Roccaforte P, Moody RA (1979) Acute intracranial hypertension and auditory brainstem responses (parts I and II). J Neurosurg 51: 669–676

35. Nagata K, Tazawa T, Mizukami M, Araki G (1984) Applications of brainstem auditory evoked potentials to evaluation of cerebral herniation. In: Nodar RH, Barber C (eds) Evoked potentials II. Butterworths Publishers, Boston, pp 183–193

36. Ottaviani F, Almadori G, Calderazzo AB, Frenguelli A, Paludetti G (1986) Auditory brain-stem and middle-latency auditory responses in the prognosis of severely head-injuries patients. Electroencephalogr Clin Neurophysiol 65: 196–202

37. Prichep LS, John ER, Ransohoff J, Cohen N, Benjamin V, Ahn H (1985) Real-time intraoperative monitoring of cranial nerves VII and VIII during posterior fossa surgery. In: Morocutti C, Rizzo PA (eds) Evoked potentials: neurophysiological and clinical aspects. Elsevier, Amsterdam, pp 193–202

38. Rosenberg C, Wogensen K, Starr A (1984) Auditory brainstem and middle and long-latency evoked potentials in coma. Arch Neurol 41: 835–838

39. Seales DM, Rossiter VS, Weinstein ME (1979) Brainstem auditory evoked responses in patients comatose as a result of blunt head trauma. J Trauma 19: 347–352

40. Sohmer H, Gafni M, Havatselet G (1984) Persistence of auditory nerve response and absence of brain-stem response in severe cerebral ischemia. Electroencephalogr Clin Neurophysiol 58: 66–72

41. Starr A (1976) Auditory brainstem responses in brain death. Brain 99: 543–554

42. Starr A, Achor J (1975) Auditory brainstem responses in neurological disease. Arch Neurol 32: 761–768

43. Starr A, Hamilton AE (1976) Correlation between confirmed sites of neurological lesions and abnormalities of far-field auditory responses. Electroencephalogr Clin Neurophysiol 41: 595–608

44. Stockard JJ, Rossiter VS (1977) Clinical and pathological correlates of brainstem auditory response abnormalities. Neurology 27: 316–325

45. Stockard JJ, Stockard JE, Sharbourgh FW (1980) Brainstem auditory evoked potentials in neurology: Methodology, interpretation, clinical application. In: Aminoff MJ (ed) Electrodiagnosis in clinical neurology. Churchill-Livingstone, New York, pp 370–413

46. Sutton LN, Frewen T, Marsh R, Jaggi J, Bruce DA (1982) The effects of deep barbiturate coma on multimodality evoked potentials. J Neurosurg 57: 178–185

47. Tsubokawa T, Nishimoto H, Yamamoto T, Kitamura M, Katayama Y, Moriyasu N (1980) Assessment of brainstem damage by the auditory brainstem response in acute severe head injury. J Neurol Neurosurg Psychiatry 43: 1005–1011

48. Uziel A, Benezech J (1978) Auditory brainstem responses in comatose patients: Relationship with brainstem reflexes and levels of coma. Electroencephalogr Clin Neurophysiol 45: 515–524

49. Walter DO (1969) "A posteriori" Wiener filtering of average evoked responses. Electroencephalogr Clin Neurophysiol [Suppl] 27: 61–70

50. De Weerd JPC, Martens WLJ (1978) Theory and practice of "a posteriori" Wiener filtering of average evoked potentials. Biol Cybernetics 30: 81–94

51. De Weerd AW, Groeneveld C (1985) The use of evoked potentials in the management of patients with severe cerebral trauma. Acta Neurol Scand 72: 489–494

Evaluation of Traumatic Coma by Means of Multimodality Evoked Potentials

M. Cenzato, A. Ducati, E. Fava*, A. Landi, E. Sganzerla, P. Baratta**, G. Signoroni**

Institute of Neurosurgery, * CNR Institute of Muscle Physiology and ** II Chair of Anesthesiology, University of Milano (Italy)

Introduction

Evoked potentials (EPs) have been used in the last several years by many authors[2, 4, 5, 8] to study comatose patients. The advantage of this technique lies in the fact that it allows an objective evaluation of neurological function in unconscious, uncooperative patients, who may be even more inaccessible to clinical assessment because of muscle relaxants or barbiturate therapy. Furthermore, this method offers the possibility of predicting outcome in comatose patients. These advantages are relevant to the treatment of patients in intensive care and rehabilitative units. Identification of the typical neurophysiological pattern of brain death is another application of this technique.

Most studies[7, 8] reported in the literature refer to patient evaluation by means of a unimodal approach only. Multimodality stimulation, exploring different pathways with different functional importance, may improve evaluation of the patient.

Patients and Methods

107 severely head-injured patients, all comatose, were studied while in the intensive care unit (ICU). Ages ranged from 5 to 68 years, with a mean age of 29; 71 patients were males, 36 females.

All patients scored 7 or less on the Glasgow Coma Scale. EPs were recorded at bedside in the ICU with commercially available systems (Amplaid MK 10 and MK 15 Multisensory System).

All data discussed here refer to the first EP records obtained, within 3 days after the traumatic event. Twenty-eight patients had EPs recorded within 6 hours of injury, and their results will be briefly discussed in the conclusions.

BAEP, short latency somatosensory EP (SSEP) and cortical late SEP (CSEP) responses were used in this study. Recording was carried out by platinum subdermal needle electrodes. Each recording was repeated at least twice in order to obtain a reliable evaluation.

BAEPs: Stimulation was with clicks of alternating polarity, 0.1 msec duration, 100 dB SPL delivered through shielded earphones to the right and left ears in separate series. White noise at an intensity 70% that of the click was simultaneously delivered to the contralateral ear.

Frequency of stimulation was either 11 or 70 pulses per second (pps), the latter in order to increase the sensitivity of the test. Filter bandwidth was 100–2,500 Hz. 2,000 sweeps were averaged over a 12 msec time base.

The interpeak latency between waves I and V and the V to I amplitude ratio were measured; these were considered abnormal when greater than 4.5 msec or less than 1 msec, respectively.

SEPs: Electrical square wave stimuli, 0.2 msec duration, were delivered to the median nerve at the wrist at an intensity exceeding three times the threshold for muscle twitch (about 20 mA).

For the *short latency SEPs* frequency of stimulation was 4 Hz. Two recording sites were used: the first one on the second cervical vertebra (SC 2) and the second over the parietal cortex (C 3′-C 4′), both referred to FpZ. 500 traces were averaged over a 30 msec analysis time. Filter bandwidth was 10–2,500 Hz. The central conduction time (CCT[5]) was calculated as the difference in latency between the cortical N 20 and the cervical N 14. Maximal CCT value accepted as normal was 6.5 msec with a maximal interhemispheric difference of 0.5 msec. For late SEPs frequency of stimulation was 1 Hz and recordings were from the parietal zone with a frontal reference. The time base was 200 msec and 100 sweeps were averaged. Filter bandwidth was 1–200 Hz.

We are aware that a midfrontal reference is currently under discussion as a possible source of mistakes in identification of wave generators. However, it has some practical advantages, mainly in reducing the biological noise that may overcome the signal (Fig. 1 A). Moreover, misinterpretation of wave generators is possible using a noncephalic reference as well, when dealing with the critically ill patient. For instance, the absence of any cortically generated activity may be evident when using a cephalic reference (Fig. 1 B), while the presence of a normal subcortical N 18, with a non-cephalic reference, may be erroneously taken for a cortical N 20. Hence, during the last year, we always used both a cephalic and noncephalic reference. To obtain homogeneous data, however, we present all our results in terms of CCT as previously defined.

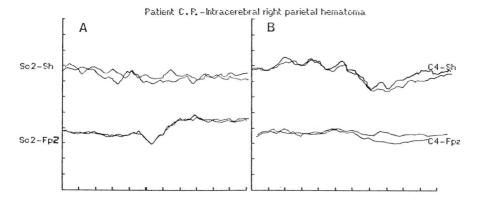

Fig. 1. Patient C.P.: persistent coma after head injury with right intracerebral parietal hematoma. Short latency traces upon left median nerve stimulation. The traces were obtained averaging 500 sweeps (with a Nicolet Pathfinder device) on a 30-msec timebase. Negativity downward. (A) *Top*: cervical recording using a noncephalic reference (contralateral shoulder). The cervical activity, if present, has been overcome by the biological noise. *Bottom*: cervical recording using a cephalic reference (FpZ). Possibly both electrodes are active and the trace is the sum of cervical and brainstem activity. However, it proves that a subcortical activity is present. (B) *Top*: cortical recording with a noncephalic reference. A large negativity is present with a latency of about 21.5 msec (possibly N 18). It could be easily interpreted as a cortical N 20 of reduced amplitude. *Bottom*: cortical recording with a cephalic reference. It is evident that no cortically generated activity is present. The C 3′ or C 4′ to FpZ montage demonstrates only cortical activity

Results

Patients were divided into 3 groups according to their BAEP response at 11 pps; SEP response allowed further subgrouping within each of these groups.

1) Normal BAEPs at 11 pps

The first group (37 patients) was characterized by a normal BAEP response at 11 pps according to the defined criteria. Clinically 15 patients had extensor responses to painful stimuli and 6 had abnormal brainstem reflexes. CT scan demonstrated, in 3 cases, hyperdensity in the upper dorsal brainstem. 26 of these patients (70%) showed an abnormal response to high frequency stimulation (70 pps). This fact suggests minor brainstem involvement even in patients with normal low frequency BAEP traces. 6 patients belonging to this group died. Among these, 4, who had an altered response at 70 pps, never regained consciousness. The other two patients died of non-neurological causes. In this group the short latency SEPs were either

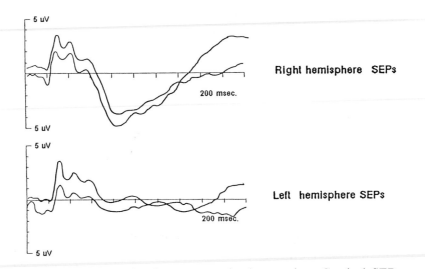

Fig. 2. Patient R.C.: left focal temporoparietal contusion. Cortical SEPs upon stimulation of the median nerve at the wrist. Negativity downward. Absence of waves following the N 20–P 25 complex is evident over the left hemisphere

normal, although close to the upper limit of normal, in 4 (10%), or altered, on one side (24, *i.e.,* 65%) or both (9, *i.e.,* 25%).

Patients showing a normal CCT also showed a normal and symmetrical N 20–P 25 complex in cortical SEPs; these all survived with a good motor outcome. Two of these patients, each with a focal contusion in the left temporoparietal area, exhibited absence of SEP late waves (the waves following the N 20–P 25 complex) on the left, even though these late waves were normally represented over the right hemisphere. Both suffered persistent aphasic disorders (Fig. 2).

Most of the patients presenting with a normal BAEP response showed a unilateral prolongation of the CCT (24 cases). These patients had a focal hemispheric lesion associated with a diffuse injury that was responsible for the comatose state.

The motor outcome of the surviving patients was more closely related to the amplitude of the N 20–P 25 cortical complex than to the CCT. 4 patients who showed a reduction in amplitude of the N 20–P 25 complex (less than 50% as compared to the contralateral side) had permanent motor disabilities. We found that cortical responses obtained with a low stimulus frequency and a longer analysis time were more reliable than short latency potentials for evaluation of amplitude.

The only 7 patients with a proven diagnosis of diffuse axonal injury were found among the patients with normal BAEP responses and bilaterally abnormal short latency SEPs. Therefore it appears that this is the typical pattern for such pathology. When followed over a period ranging from six months to three years, these patients all had moderate disability according to the Glasgow Outcome Scale.

2) Complete but Abnormal BAEPs

41 patients showed an altered but complete BAEP response; *i.e.,* even though the I–V interpeak latency was prolonged, all waves were present. It is necessary to stress that in this series the responses were never pathological on one side only; despite different degrees of involvement, both sides were affected.

All patients showed extensor responses to painful stimuli. 23 patients had pathological brainstem reflexes and 18 had asymmetric motor responses. In 4 cases respiratory failure was present. CT scan demonstrated hemispheric lesions without signs of direct brainstem involvement in 21 cases, while in 9 cases either brainstem hemorrhage or absence of basal cisterns was evident. 21 patients belonging to this group died (51%). Patients who had bilateral short latency SEP alterations also had a high mortality rate; 17 of 28 patients with bilateral prolongation died (60%). In contrast only 4 of the 13 patients with unilateral CCT prolongation died (30%).

A unilateral alteration of short latency SEPs associated with bilateral alterations of BAEPs, can be ascribed to a supratentorial lesion with secondary effects on the brainstem. In this case, the prognosis is mainly related to the evolution of supratentorial lesion and the secondary brainstem damage.

A pattern characterized by bilaterally altered BAEPs associated with bilateral prolongation of CCT on SEP responses is generally due to multiple supratentorial lesions with secondary brainstem involvement. In one case, however, BAEPs showed a normal wave V amplitude while the I-V interpeak latency (ipl) was prolonged. This pattern suggests a specific brainstem lesion below the mesencephalic level that can also be responsible for the bilateral CCT prolongation.

3) Absent BAEPs Bilaterally

The 29 patients in this group were characterized by incomplete BAEP traces (Fig. 3). It was never possible to identify waves IV and V, while wave I was always visible. Clinically all these patients showed decerebrate responses, pathological brainstem reflexes, and respiratory failure. CT scan always demonstrated either a hemorrhagic lesion or undetectable cisterns. Short latency SEP traces showed a bilateral CCT prolongation up to 11 msec; but in 17 cases the cortical N 20 was undetectable and, conse-

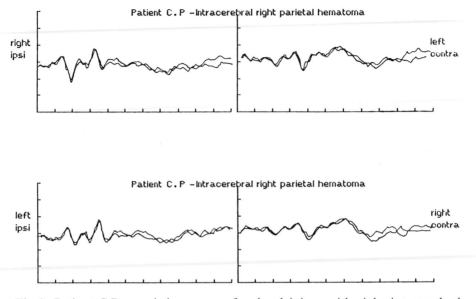

Fig. 3. Patient C.P.: persisting coma after head injury with right intracerebral parietal hematoma. Typical BAEP pattern characterized by bilateral absence of peaks following the wave III

quently, CCT was not measurable. The mortality rate of this group was 100%. Hence, the bilaterally incomplete BAEP response is the worst prognostic sign. The typical pattern of brain death is the presence of BAEP wave I, and of the SEP cervical N 14, bilaterally, in the absence of any following, previously seen, activity generated in the brainstem or in the cortex. When this pattern appears, an irreversible brainstem lesion has taken place.

Conclusions

Evaluation of comatose patients by means of multimodality evoked potentials makes the diagnostic and prognostic assessment more precise, especially in the acute phase.

The limitation of the technique is that it has a very low specificity, in spite of a high sensitivity. Hence, an etiological diagnosis is never possible. From a practical point of view, the effects on EPs of previous or associated pathologies, such as multiple sclerosis or severe metabolic derangements, are not distinguishable from the consequence of head trauma. However, when EP data are integrated into a complete clinical evaluation of the patient, diagnostic accuracy is higher than that obtainable from either the Glasgow Coma Scale[6] or the measurement of intracranial pressure (ICP)[1].

As shown in Fig. 4, the outcomes of our patients differed markedly

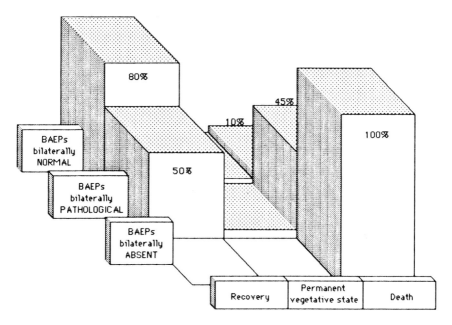

Fig. 4. Outcome of patients according to the three groups of BAEP traces as described in the text

among the groups defined according to the BAEP findings. Unlike other authors[3] we do not believe that a I to V IPL longer than 4.48 msec invariably leads either to death or to a permanent vegetative state (PVS). The only pattern of EPs that was invariably associated with death in our series was an incomplete BAEP response. BAEPs are not appropriate for forecasting PVS, since this syndrome is caused mainly by diffuse cortical injury with a still functioning brainstem. PVS may be found, as in our series, among patients with either normal or abnormal BAEPs; the common characteristic of PVS patients is absence of severe reduction of the cortical SEP response. This particular result stresses the importance of a multimodality EP study for an optimal evaluation of head-injured patients.

We believe that the use of a frontal reference for SEP recordings has definite advantages when recording is done in the ICU, particularly in a patient with decerebrate activity. Meaningful results are always obtainable with a frontal reference, as long as it is recognized that no precise identification of subcortical wave generators is possible. On the other hand, a frontal reference is required to identify with certainty pure cortical activity; this distinction may be difficult in the critically ill patient, when only a noncephalic reference is used. In our experience, the best methodological approach is to use both a cephalic and noncephalic reference.

Finally, when BAEP responses were recorded within six hours of head injury, only 1 of 28 patients presented with an abnormal response. This patient had a trace compatible with a primary brainstem lesion, *i.e.,* a prolonged I to V interpeak latency but a normal amplitude of wave V. This means that a very large majority of brainstem abnormalities are secondary to hemispheric lesions. Aggressive and effective treatment might, therefore, reduce the devastating effects of this traumatic pathology.

References

1. Anderson DC, Bundlie S, Rockswould GL (1984) Multimodality evoked potentials in close head trauma. Arch Neurol 41: 369–374
2. Ducati A, Parmeggiani F, Antonelli A, Villani R (1983) Early evaluation of prognosis using BAEPs in patients with post-traumatic disorders of consciousness. In: Villani R, Papo I, Giovanelli M, Gaini SM, Tomei G (eds) Advances in neurotraumatology, International Series 612, Excerpta Medica, Amsterdam Oxford Princeton, pp 214–218
3. Facco E, Martini A, Zuccarello M, Agnoletto M, Giron GP (1985) Is the auditory evoked brainstem response (ABR) effective in the assessment of post-traumatic coma? Electroencephalogr Clin Neurophysiol 62: 332–337
4. Greenberg RP, Becker DP, Miller JD, Mayer DJ (1977) Evaluation of brainstem conduction in severe head trauma with multimodality evoked potentials. J Neurosurg 47: 163–167
5. Hume AC, Cant BR (1981) Central somatosensory conduction time after head injury. Ann Neurol 10: 411–419
6. Karnaze DS, Weiner JM, Marshall LF (1985) Auditory evoked potentials in coma after closed head injury: a clinical-neurophysiologic coma scale for predicting outcome. Neurology 35: 1122–1126
7. Klug N (1982) Brainstem auditory evoked potentials in syndromes of decerebration, the bulbar syndrome and in central death. J Neurol 227: 219–228
8. Lindslay KW, Carlin J, Kennedy I, Fry J, McInness A, Teasdale GM (1981) Evoked Potentials in severe head injury: analysis and relation to outcome. J Neurol Neurosurg Psychiatry 44: 796–802
9. Rumpl E, Prugger M, Gerstenbrand F, Hackl JM, Paulla A (1983) Central somatosensory conduction time and short latency somatosensory evoked potentials in post-traumatic coma. Electroencephalogr Clin Neurophysiol 56: 583–596

Intraoperative Monitoring of Cortical and Spinal Evoked Potentials Using Different Stimulation Sites

E. Watanabe, J. Schramm, J. Romstöck

University of Erlangen-Nürnberg (Federal Republic of Germany)

Introduction

In spinal cord monitoring spinal and cortical recording techniques may be used[1, 2, 3, 4, 5, 7]. In addition different stimulation sites have also been used: peripheral nerves, cauda equina or the dorsal surface of the spinal cord[8, 9, 11, 12]. Whether cortical or spinal recordings are superior is not yet settled. It is also unknown whether the use of invasive stimulation sites, *i.e.,* the cauda equina, will give more reliable and thus more useful recordings than peripheral nerve stimulation. Therefore, in our current series of spinal cord monitoring during operations on space occupying lesions we compared different stimulation sites as often as possible.

Patients and Methods

During the last two years we monitored more than 50 cases during neurosurgical procedures; 40 cases were analyzed for this presentation. There were 15 cervical lesions, 18 thoracic and 7 lumbar. The diagnoses were meningioma (12 cases), syringomyelia (4 cases), neurinoma (2 cases) and 15 miscellaneous lesions including ependymoma and metastasis. We did not include any operations for trauma or spinal deformity.

Stimulation: The stimulus was a constant current square wave of 200–300 μsec duration, delivered transcutaneously via conventional paired skin electrodes to the peroneal nerve in the popliteal fossa or the median nerve at the wrist. For cauda equina stimulation a conventional 16-G lumbar puncture needle was used to perform lumbar puncture and the second electrode was usually a paramedian subcutaneous needle. Stimulation strength in the preoperative recordings usually was enough to elect a muscle twitch, or at least three times sensory threshold.

During anesthesia and operation we usually increased the stimulating

Table 1. *Stimulus Site*

Lesion site	Median nerve	Peroneal nerve	Cauda equina
15 cervical	15	13	2
18 thoracic	12	17	15
7 lumbar	0	7	1

current to 20 mA. Stimulation frequency was 5.3 Hz for cortical recording, between 5.3 and 50 Hz for epidural recording. A constant current stimulator was used.

Recording: A 4-channel Nicolet CA 1000 system was used. For each average 200–300 sweeps were sufficient; the bandpass of the amplifier was 30–3,000 Hz (in a few cases 30–1,500 Hz). The automatic artifact rejection of the CA 1000 was always used; in case of severe artifacts due to electrocautery of the ultrasonic aspirator, monitoring was manually interrupted.

After induction of anesthesia recording was usually started with scalp (C 3,4 or Cz-Fz) and spinal skin (Cv 7-Fz; T 12-Fz) electrodes. As soon as the dura was exposed, a pair of monopolar recording electrodes (diameter 1 mm) was placed on the dura over the dorsal surface of the cord above and below the lesion. The reference electrode was located on the scalp (Fz). Recordings were obtained continuously throughout the operation, alternating among the different stimulation sites. In some patients it was not possible to compare two stimulation sites (Table 1). In these patients we also used different recording sites, usually with simultaneous recording at different levels[3, 9].

Evaluation of recordings: The traces were classified as either unobtainable or useful according to their reproducibility.

Unobtainable recordings were those in which no reproducible waves were found. Useful recordings were those in which the peaks could always be easily defined with good reproducibility, this group included all cases with some degree of transient change and increased variability compared with the stable group. Cases with marked intraoperative changes in evoked potentials (improvement, deterioration, or loss), which would be included in the useful group, are not discussed in this report.

Results

Comparison in Same Patient

In Tables 2 and 3 the usefulness and quality of cortical recordings obtained after using two different stimulation sites in the *same* patient are compared. In 12 *cervical lesions,* median nerve stimulation and peroneal nerve stim-

Table 2. *Quality and Reproducibility of Cortical Potentials in Median versus Peroneal Nerve Stimulation*

12 cervical lesions	
Med > Peron	4
Med = Peron	7
Med < Peron	1

Table 3. *Quality and Reproducibility of Cortical Potentials in Cauda Equina versus Peroneal Nerve Stimulation*

16 thoracolumbar lesions	
Cauda > Peron	4
Cauda = Peron	10
Cauda < Peron	2

ulation were alternatingly used in the same patient. As can be seen in Table 2 the quality and reproducibility of the cortical potentials after peroneal nerve stimulation was judged to be better in just one case. In the majority of cases (N = 7) the quality was equal, while the cortical potentials after median nerve stimulation were better and more useful than peroneal nerve potentials in four cases. Thus for cervical lesions, median nerve stimulation served our purpose at least as well as peroneal nerve stimulation in 11 out of 12 cases, whereas peroneal nerve stimulation was superior to median nerve stimulation in just one case.

In 16 *thoraco-lumbar lesions* (all of them affecting the cord, not the cauda equina) peroneal nerve stimulation and cauda equina stimulation were used alternately in the same patient. The quality of the *cortical* recordings was similar in 10 of these 16 cases. Potentials after cauda equina stimulation were superior to peroneal nerve stimulation in 4 cases, but peroneal nerve evoked potentials were superior to cauda equina evoked potentials in two cases. It follows that for thoracic spinal cord lesions, cauda equina stimulation or peroneal nerve stimulation may be used with a similar chance of achieving satisfactory potentials. Since obtaining these results we usually use peroneal nerve recordings and only add cauda equina stimulation when the position of the patient and the draping allow this technique.

In a subgroup of 6 patients epidural recordings were compared after cauda equina stimulation and after peroneal nerve stimulation in the *same* patient. The epidural recordings caudal to the lesion were of the same quality in 5 of these 6 patients; in one case we were unable to obtain a good potential with cauda equina stimulation for technical reasons (inadequate placing of the stimulus needle). The epidural recording above the lesion was of the same quality in all 6 patients, but in one of the cases the configuration of the recording with cauda equina stimulation was different, showing an "evoked injury potential", whereas the potential after peroneal nerve stimulation showed a normally configured triphasic potential. Thus, for epidural recordings, no significant differences could be detected between cauda equina and peroneal nerve stimulation concerning the *quality* of recordings. In one case, however, more information was obtained from the *wave form* with cauda equina stimulation.

Cumulative Results

Unobtainable recordings: Table 4 shows the percentage of unobtainable recordings grouped for different stimulation sites and recording sites. Technically speaking, the percentage of unobtainable recordings, for whatever reason, represents the number of technical failures. Since recordings were performed at several levels (L 5-skin, T 12-skin, T 4/5-skin, C 7-skin, scalp and epidurally) the sum of all recordings in all patients obtained after stimulating the peroneal nerve is larger than the number of patients in whom that recording mode was used. Contrary to the results given in Tables 2 and 3, the figures given in Tables 4 and 5 summarize *all* recordings and no differentiation has been made among the different recording sites. Therefore it is possible to compare the number of unobtainable recordings following stimulation at different sites. It can be seen that the percentage of unobtainable recordings is lowest after median nerve stimulation. It is also evident that recordings were more often useful below than above the

Table 4. *Unobtainable Recordings*

Stimulation site	Above the lesion			Below the lesion		
	N	Sum all recordings	%	N	Sum all recordings	%
Peroneal nerve	11	75	15	1	31	3
Median nerve	2	23	9	1	15	7
Cauda equina	11	40	28	3	12	25

Table 5. *Useful Recordings*

Stimulation site	Above the lesion			Below the lesion		
	N	Sum all recordings	%	N	Sum all recordings	%
Peroneal nerve	64	75	85	30	31	97
Median nerve	21	23	91	14	15	93
Cauda equina	29	40	72	9	12	75

lesion. The most remarkable finding is the high percentage of unobtainable recordings following cauda equina stimulation. This will be discussed later.

Useful recordings: Table 5 shows the percentages of stable recordings following median nerve, peroneal nerve, and cauda equina stimulation, summarizing all the recording sites above and below the lesion. The lowest proportion of useful recordings was obtained after cauda equina stimulation. After median nerve and peroneal nerve stimulation, 93% and 97% of recordings, respectively, were useful. It should be noted that the group of useful recordings contained several subgroups, including those cases with significant intraoperative changes to better or worse and also those cases in which an evoked injury potential was obtained in the epidural recording site. No specification has been made for the different recording sites, but the quality of recording sometimes varied remarkably from one site to the other.

Discussion

When discussing our results some remarks should be made on the invasiveness of cauda equina stimulation. We do not consider cauda equina stimulation to be more invasive than the arterial puncture, which in many cases is used by the anesthesiologist in treating these patients during surgery. In neurosurgical tumor cases the subarachnoid space will be opened in most cases anyway, so the potential risk of introduction of infection into the subarachnoid space is not so avoidable as in orthopedic cases. We believe that no additional harm is added by inserting a needle into the subarachnoid space in these cases where the dura is open, sometimes for several hours.

From the experience of other authors no particular mention has been made concerning risks of this method[5, 7, 8, 12, 13, 14]. Other authors in the meantime have used different spinal recording techniques[3, 4] and tried to avoid introduction of an electrode into the subarachnoid space but could not because of the poor quality of spinal potentials recorded from the

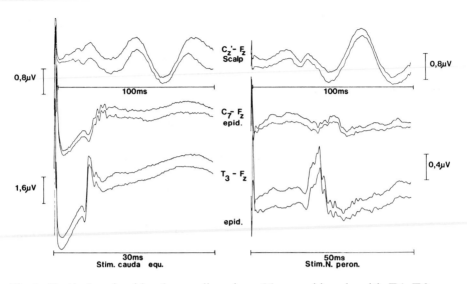

Fig. 1. Cortical and epidural recordings in a 56-year-old male with T1–T2 meningioma. The waveform above the lesion is altered compared with the recording
below. Cortical potentials are normal. Note differing analysis times, positivity is
shown downward (from ref.[8])

skin. Our findings (not described in this paper) also showed a very high
figure for unobtainable recordings when using skin recordings.

Our results comparing two different stimulation sites in the same patient
indicate quite clearly that, in cervical lesions, median nerve stimulation
seems superior to peroneal nerve stimulation. This may be explained by
several causes. First, the number of fibers in the cervical cord originating
in the median nerve is much larger than the number of fibers from the
peroneal nerve. It is well known that, due to branching, at least 35% of
all fibers from the lower extremity never reach the dorsal column nuclei[6].
Another reason may be that our patients with cervical lesions were less
affected by the lesion than the group of patients with thoraco-lumbar
lesions, although from the degree of neurological change we did not have
this impression. For planning a monitoring procedure, however, one can
decide to use median nerve stimulation primarily in cervical lesions.

In thoraco-lumbar lesions none of the two stimulus sites showed particular advantage. It should be noted that there is a difference between
spinal recordings and cortical recordings when considering cauda equina
stimulation in patients with these lesions. On the one hand, if the lesion
is situated rather low, the stimulus artifact from cauda equina stimulation
may interfere with spinal recordings. This is the factor responsible for the

high number of unobtainable recordings below the lesion after cauda equina stimulation shown in Table 4. In a previous study comparing the variability of latencies and amplitudes of *cortical* potentials[10] we pointed out that these potentials were more stable after cauda equina stimulation than after peroneal nerve stimulation. On the other hand, in some cases we could not obtain good cortical potentials at all with peroneal nerve stimulation but we saw good potentials after stimulation of the cauda equina. The relatively high proportion of unobtainable recordings after cauda equina stimulation (Table 4) must not lead to the conclusion that cauda equina stimulation is useless, because marked differences between the two stimulation sites are possible from patient to patient. Table 3 shows that in 4 of 16 cases cauda equina stimulation was better than peroneal nerve stimulation. Thus when planning a monitor procedure for a thoracic tumor (especially a low lying

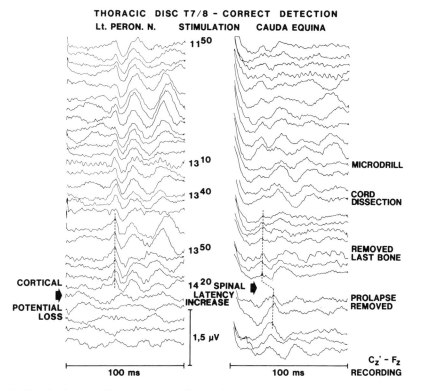

Fig. 2. Cortical recordings after cauda equina versus peroneal nerve stimulation in a case with T 6/7 thoracic disc operation. The potential recorded after peroneal nerve stimulation showed a sudden amplitude decrease when the thoracic disc prolapse was removed from the spinal canal and pulled back into the disc space. Note at the same moment, the potential after cauda equina stimulation showed latency elongation rather than amplitude decrease. This patient showed a persistent worsening of neurologic status after surgery

thoracic tumor) one can use either method of stimulation but should be prepared to use the other technique if the first method fails.

No significant advantages of epidural recordings were detected in our small group of 6 patients. In one case, however, we obtained information with stimulation of the cauda equina, that we could not obtain by using peroneal nerve stimulation: the wave configuration showed a so-called "evoked injury potential". The most likely reason for this is that stimulation of the peroneal nerve activated fewer fibers, especially fibers unimpaired by the spinal cord tumor, so that the epidural recording after peroneal nerve stimulation looked normal. With cauda equina stimulation more fibers were activated, including those that were compressed by the tumor, producing the "evoked injury potential". Theoretically speaking, cauda equina stimulation might give better information because more fibers are involved. On the other hand, when using cauda equina stimulation one gives up the advantage of comparing the potentials generated when the right and the left peroneal nerves are stimulated separately. The importance of this comparison has been pointed out by Maccabee *et al.*[3]. The number of fibers may also explain the different potential changes after cauda equina and peroneal nerve stimulation in Fig. 2. The loss of potential occurred only after stimulation of the left peroneal nerve.

Our results show that the quality of potentials obtained both at spinal and cortical levels is influenced not only by the stimulation site (and many other technical factors), but also to a significant degree by the presence of a lesion. It has also been pointed out by others[9, 12] that the presence of a spinal cord lesion, be it traumatic or space occupying, is important for the monitoring procedure.

Summary

The quality of somatosensory evoked potentials following stimulation at different sites for intraoperative spinal cord monitoring was assessed. We found that for cervical lesions median nerve stimulation was preferable to stimulation of the peroneal nerve. In thoraco-lumbar cord lesions either peroneal nerve stimulation or cauda equina stimulation gave approximately the same results. In those cases where the peripheral stimulation site gave unsatisfactory results, cauda equina stimulation sometimes produced better waveforms. In one case, cauda equina stimulation provided more information than peroneal nerve stimulation, because an "evoked injury potential" was demonstrable only when the cauda equina was stimulated.

References

1. Jones SJ, Carter L, Edgar MA, Morley T, Ransford AO, Webb PJ (1985) Experience of epidural spinal cord monitoring in 410 cases. In: Schramm J, Jones SJ (eds) Spinal cord monitoring. Springer, Berlin Heidelberg New York, pp 215–220

2. Koht A, Sloan T, Ronai A, Toleikis JR (1985) Intraoperative deterioration of evoked potentials during spinal surgery. In: Schramm J, Jones SJ (eds) Spinal cord monitoring. Springer, Berlin Heidelberg New York, pp 161–166

3. Maccabee PJ, Levine DB, Pinkhasov EI, Cracco RQ, Tsairis P (1983) Evoked potentials recorded from scalp and spinous processes during spinal column surgery. Electroencephalogr Clin Neurophysiol 56: 569–582

4. Macon JB, Poletti CE, Sweet WH, Ojemann RG, Zervas N (1982) Conducted somatosensory evoked potentials during spinal surgery. Part 2: Clinical applications. J Neurosurg 57: 354–359

5. Maruyama Y, Shimizu H, Fujioka H et al (1984) Spinal cord function monitoring by spinal cord potentials during spine and spinal surgery. In: Homma S, Tamaki T (eds) Fundamentals and clinical application of spinal cord monitoring. Tokio, Saikon, pp 191–202

6. Norton AC, Kruger L (1973) The dorsal column system of the spinal cord. Its anatomy, physiology, phylogeny and sensory function. An updated review, ed 5. Los Angeles: UCLA Brain Information Service, pp 62–73, 108–122

7. Ohmi Y, Tohno S, Harata S, Nakano K (1984) Spinal cord monitoring using evoked potentials recorded from epidural space. In: Homma S, Tamaki T (eds) Fundamentals and clinical application of spinal cord monitoring. Tokio, Saikon, pp 203–210

8. Schramm J (1985) Spinal cord monitoring: Current status and new developments. CNS Trauma 2: 207–227

9. Schramm J (1986) Intraoperative spinal cord monitoring. Adv Neurosurg 14: 17–21

10. Schramm J, Romstöck J, Thurner F, Fahlbusch R (1985) Variance of latencies and amplitudes in SEP monitored during operations with and without cord manipulation. In: Schramm J, Jones SJ (eds) Spinal cord monitoring. Springer, Berlin Heidelberg New York, pp 186–196

11. Takano H, Tamaki T, Noguchi T, Takakuwa K (1985) Comparison of spinal cord evoked potentials elicited by spinal cord and peripheral nerve stimulation. In: Schramm J, Jones SJ (eds) Spinal cord monitoring. Springer, Berlin Heidelberg New York, pp 29–34

12. Tamaki T, Takano H, Takakuwa K, Tsuji H, Nakagawa T, Imai K, Inoue S (1985) An assessment of the use of spinal cord evoked potentials in prognosis estimation of injured spinal cord. In: Schramm J, Jones SJ (eds) Spinal cord monitoring. Springer, Berlin Heidelberg New York, pp 221–226

13. Whittle IR, Johnston IH, Besser M (1984) Spinal cord monitoring during surgery by direct recording of somatosensory evoked potentials. J Neurosurg 60: 440–443

14. Whittle IR, Johnston IH, Besser M (1986) Intraoperative recording of cortical somatosensory evoked potential as a method of spinal cord monitoring during spinal surgery. Aust NZJ Surg 56: 309–317

Radicular Somatosensory Evoked Potentials Recording During Foraminotomy

A. Pansini, G. De Luca, P. Conti, R. Conti, F. Lo Re, P. Bono, P. Gallina, G. Pellicano'

Department of Neurosurgery, University of Firenze (Italy)

Summary

Among the various cerebral and myeloradicular pathologies in which we use a BASIS EPM for somatosensory evoked potential (SEP) recording, we have given much attention to the study of the cervical radicular compressions.

The motor and sensory alterations are evidenced by means of the electromyographic (EMG) and electroneurographic (ENG) methods, allowing a fine analysis of the function of these systems at distal and proximal parts of the nerve, including the metameric spinal cord.

SEPs offer the advantage of verifying the transmission of the sensory stimulus leading to the cortex.

The use of SEPs in the pre- and postsurgical phases, associated with EMG and ENG, has allowed us to demonstrate the amplitude, morphology and latency of the evoked responses at various levels, supplying the necessary data on the functional status of the sensory systems near the lesion. Together with the clinical and neuroradiological findings, the SEP has allowed us to follow the evolution of the disease and to verify and determine the degree of the effectiveness of the surgical intervention.

We recently initiated intraoperative recording of the SEP to immediately verify the restoration of radicular conduction at the intervertebral foramen level with special flexible metal hooked electrodes that are directly inserted on the nerve root and needle electrodes placed at Erb's point and on other recording points.

If the sensory conduction at the intervertebral foramen level, which has been widened by means of foraminotomy, is well restored, an evoked response obtained by means of peripheral electric stimulation shows a far greater amplitude than all other responses.

By analyzing the latency, amplitude, morphology and timing of this response, and comparing these parameters with others, we obtain an immediate verification of the effectiveness of the operation.

Introduction

In the neurosurgical management of myeloradicular pathology, we have, during recent years, concentrated on compressions from arthrotic spurs at the cervical level.

This kind of pathology produces a large variety of symptomatic pictures, including medial compressions of spinal cord due to herniated disc or marginal posteromedial osteophytes; radicular compressions due to side disc herniation or arthrotic spurs, which reduce the amplitude of the intervertebral foramen; and all the symptom of the myeloradicular compression with different clinical manifestations. The variety of clinical syndromes may easily lead to incorrect diagnosis.

In order to reach a proper surgical decision based on correct diagnosis, we use a neuroradiological protocol including the following tests: roentgenograms in the anteroposterior, lateral and oblique right and left projections, with hyperflexion and hyperextension; laminograms; myelography; high resolution computerized tomography (CT) scan; CT myelography; tridimensional CT reconstruction of the intervertebral foramen; magnetic resonance imaging (MRI).

We also make a functional evaluation with EMG and electroneurographic (ENG) methods and, recently, with SEPs. The evolution of EMG methods today makes it possible to test the function of the peripheral motor and sensory nerves and the corresponding metameric spinal cord. The SEPs allow a detailed analysis of the conduction of the somatosensory stimulus at both peripheral and central levels, up to the somatosensory area of the cerebral cortex.

These diagnostic methods confirm the results of neuroradiological studies.

By combining the morphological and functional results with the history and physical examination, it is possible to formulate a correct diagnosis and reach a correct surgical decision for a median longitudinal corpectomy, a laminectomy with foraminotomy or a laminectomy alone. The corpectomy, a surgical technique first developed by our school, is performed when there is an anterior medullar compression. The foraminotomy is specifically carried out for radicular compression at the intervertebral foramen level. The laminectomy is still used when the disease caused by a stenosis concerns the anterior and posterior spinal cord structures.

Material and Methods

To perform SEP and EMG we use a 4-channel commercial instrument (Biopotential Analyzer Software Interactive System for Evoked Potentials and Myography, BASIS EPM, OTE Biomedica Elettronica of Florence,

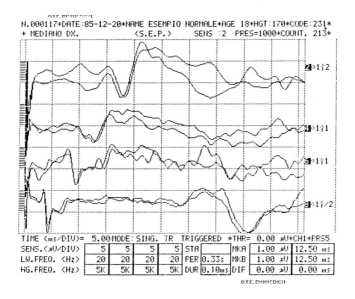

Fig. 1. Normal subject. From bottom to top evoked responses: elbow, Erb's point, CV–VI, somatosensory cortex

Italy) with the following technical properties: 8 traces of 1,024 points each sampled at a velocity of 2 µs per point; videographic memory with a capacity of 131,072 points; averager with memory of 4,096 points for 20 bits; a wide oscilloscope screen (12″); a magnetic floppy disk unit; somatosensory, auditory and visual (flash and pattern reversal) stimulators completely managed and controlled via software.

We use the parameters supplied by the Italian Society of EEG and Clinical Neurophysiology to record the SEP: time base 5 ms/div, sensitivity 5 µV/div, filters 20–5,000 Hz, stimulus frequency 3 Hz, stimulus duration 0.1 ms, and intensity of stimulation 50–100 V (up to evident distal motor responses) and stimulation of median nerve at wrist, 200–1,000 stimulations; derivations at elbow, Erb's point, CV–VI, and somatosensory cortex (C 3′-C 4′); and frontal reference (FpZ). In normal subjects the use of such a system allows very clear and adequately reproducible evoked responses (Fig. 1).

According to the clinical and neuroradiological findings, we can stimulate the ulnar or radial nerve; also, we can stimulate the axilla or Erb's point.

For about 3 years we have been recording the SEP and EMG on both sides preoperatively in order to find out the level of the disease and measure the neuronal damage[2, 3]. The tests performed either shortly after the operation or later on helped us formulate an exact prognosis and verify the

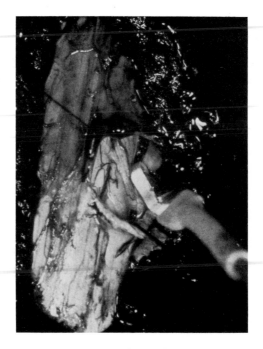

Fig. 2. The electrode on the nerve root

results of surgical treatment. We have considered it very important to record SEP during the operation to obtain immediate confirmation that the surgical intervention was successful, especially in presence of neuronal damage due to compression at the intervertebral foramen. This is accomplished by recording the evoked responses both before and after decompression. During the operation the evoked responses are recorded with a common needle electrode at Erb's point and a flexible flat electrode on the nerve root (Fig. 2). The common reference is placed on FpZ^{1-4}.

Case Reports

The above method, still under development, has been applied in the following 2 cases:

Patient 1: A 50-year-old female, admitted on Sept. 2, 1985, had suffered 15 years from cervical pain which increased over time. For the 18 months before admission, she had weakness, slight difficulty with finger movements, hypesthesia, and dysesthesia mainly affecting the distal right arm. For a few months, she had similar symptoms of the right leg and slight sphincter dysfunction.

Clinical examinations showed atrophy of the first interosseous muscle, weakness when she closed her hand tight, and when using two fingers,

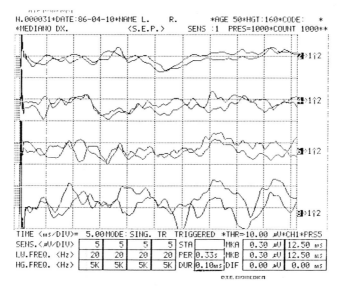

O.T.E. BIOMEDICA

Fig. 3

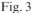

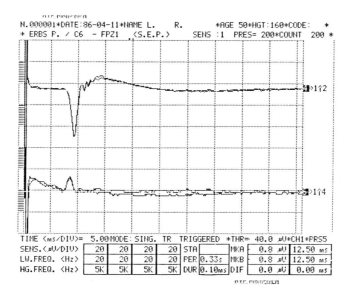

O.T.E. BIOMEDICA

Fig. 4

global hypesthesia of C 6, C 7, and C 8, and hyperreflexia of the right arm and leg.

Lumbar puncture showed clear colorless cerebrospinal fluid, with total proteins 0.32 g/l and one cell. Roentgenograms showed reduced physiological lordosis, an abnormal disc at CV–VI, and arthrosis affecting the

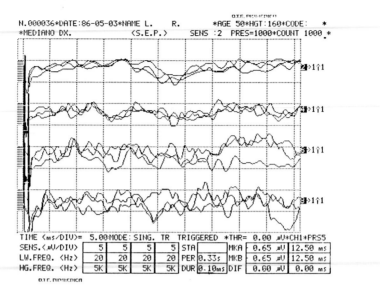

Fig. 5

uncinate processes at CV–VI. Myelography showed an anterior compression at CV–VI that was more evident in hyperextension. CT-myelography showed arthrosis of vertebral margins even posteriorly with marked impression on the dura mater, particularly at the CV–VI level, with bilateral stenosis of intervertebral foramina. Tridimensional CT showed marked stenosis of intervertebral foramina at the CV–VI level. MRI showed marked backward displacement of CV–VI with impression on the dura mater, but no disc herniation. On preoperative SEP, evoked responses had normal latencies but did not replicate very well (Fig. 3).

Posterior laminectomy was done from CV to VII and extended on right side foraminotomy to release the C 6 root which was compressed by a bony protrusion. After the dura mater was opened an electrode was placed on the nerve root. Intraoperative SEP showed a prominent radicular evoked response with amplitude greater than 25 µV with a peak at 9 msec. The evoked response at Erb's point had an amplitude of 7–8 µV with a peak at 8 msec latency (Fig. 4).

After the operation there was a rapid progressive reduction of the pain and paresthesia, which disappeared completely in 15 days. The patient showed excellent improvement in motor function, and sphincter function returned to normal. Postoperative SEP recordings showed prominent evoked responses with normal latency and improved replication, but cortical responses showed low voltage (Fig. 5).

Patient 2: A 55-year-old man was admitted on April 3, 1986. For 15 years the patient had suffered from progressive cervical pain. For two years

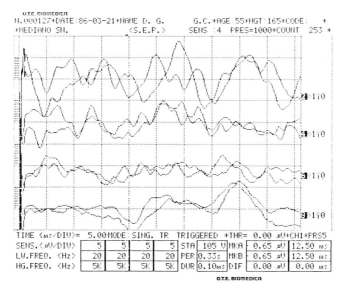

Fig. 6

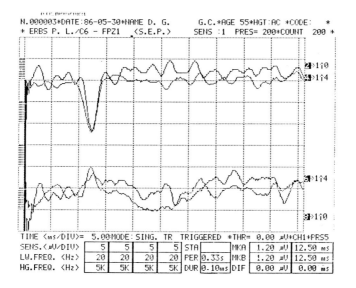

Fig. 7

the patient had pain and paresthesia in the left arm and in the first three fingers of the left hand. He complained of progressive weakness in left arm and slight sphincter dysfunction. Clinical examination showed reduced mobility of the neck and difficulty in finger movement with marked weakness when using two fingers. There was marked atrophy of the first inter-

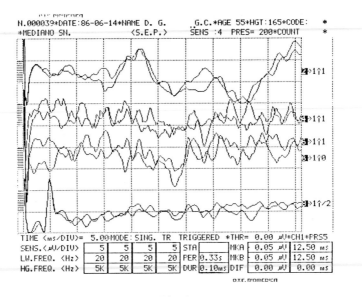

Fig. 8

osseous muscle and hypesthesia in the distributions of C5, C6, and C7 on the left side. Hyperreflexia was also present in the left arm.

Roentgenograms showed evident intersomatic arthrosis in CV–VI with bilateral neurocentral osteophytes, particularly on the left side and foraminal stenosis at CV–VI and CVI–VII, particularly on the left side. Myelography showed a block at CV–VI. Oblique projections confirmed that the left side showed more damage. CT demonstrated marked arthrosis of the vertebral margin and confirmed the foraminal stenosis. On MRI several impressions on the dura mater were evident, more marked anteriorly and at intervertebral discs. Preoperative SEPs were not identified either at the elbow or at the cortical level. Questionable responses with poor superimposition were seen at Erb's point and CVI, with normal latency. The Erb's point response was hardly visible (Fig. 6). Laminectomy was performed at CV and CVI, extended on the left side and foraminotomy was done at C6 level. The nerve root showed backward compression due to a prominent body protrusion.

An electrode was applied on the sheath of the nerve root. Intraoperative SEP showed evoked responses at left Erb's point of 2 μV amplitude and 12.2 msec latency with even more prominent radicular responses of 3 μV amplitude and 12.2 ms latency (Fig. 7).

After the operation there was a rapid improvement in hand movement. Pain, weakness, and sphincter dysfunction disappeared in about 15 days. SEPs done 15 days after operation replicated well and were much more clearly defined than the preoperative responses. Particularly at the elbow and at the cortical level, responses were clear, with normal amplitude, morphology and latency (Fig. 8).

Conclusions

Because the recording of intraoperative SEP has been used only recently, it would be premature to draw definite conclusions; nevertheless, we believe we have developed an extremely useful method for immediate verification of the effects of foraminotomy.

Analysis of radicular evoked potentials will allow a better interpretation of single components of cervical responses, especially if we extend this analysis to the responses recorded from the dorsal columns in cervical cord.

Finally, we plan to apply such a method to investigation of the motor roots, by using either direct stimulation or transcutaneous cortical stimulation[5].

References

1. Aki T, Toya S (1984) Experimental study on changes of the spinal evoked potential and circulatory dynamics following spinal cord compression and decompression. Spine 9 (8): 800–809
2. D'Alpa F, Russo T, Bonfiglio G, Pero G, Grasso A (1985) Assessment of spinal cord conduction in cervical myelopathies by spinal stenosis or herniated disc. Acta Neurol (Napoli) 7 (5): 394–400
3. Emerson RG, Pedley TA (1986) Effect of cervical spinal cord lesions on early components of the median nerve somatosensory evoked potentials. Neurology 36 (1): 20–26
4. Keim HA, Haydu M, Gonzalez EG, Brand L, Balasubramanian E (1985) Somatosensory evoked potentials as an aid in the diagnosis and intraoperative management of spinal stenosis. Spine 10 (4): 338–344
5. Machida M, Weinstein SL, Yamada T, Kimura J (1985) Spinal cord monitoring: electrophysiological measures of sensory and motor function during spinal surgery. Spine 10 (5): 407–413

1987. 133 partly colored figures.
X, 289 pages.
Cloth DM 220,—, öS 1540,—
ISBN 3-211-81987-8

Contents: Introduction — Acute Ischemic Neurological Deficits: AINDs — Delayed Ischemic Neurological Deficits: DINDs — Relevance of the Metabolism of Membrane Lipids to Cerebral Vasospasm and Ischemic Brain Damage — Grading of Risk, Angiography and Computerized Tomography — Surgical Indications and Decision Making — Perioperative Care — Surgical Techniques — Résumé.

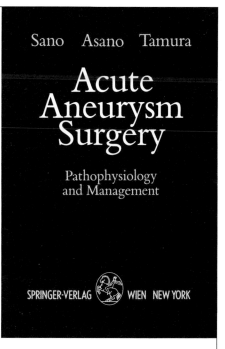

Sano Asano Tamura

Acute Aneurysm Surgery

Pathophysiology and Management

SPRINGER-VERLAG WIEN NEW YORK

During the recent years, major advances in surgical techniques, diagnostic methods, anesthesia and adjunctive treatment in the care of patients with subarachnoid hemorrhage have been achieved. Still, the overall outcome of patients with SAH cannot be regarded as satisfactory.

The first part of the book concentrates on the pathogenetic machanisms underlying vasospasm and edema, which are the principle causes of poor outcome. Recent progress in the field of membrane lipid metabolism has allowed to approach the problem from an entirely new aspect. The possible participation of free radicals, membrane lipids and eicosanoids are thoroughly discussed.

The second part features the problems of practical management of SAH patients: Timing and indication of surgery of aneurysms and the surgical techniques are described in detail.

Springer-Verlag Wien New York

Moelkerbastei 5, A-1010 Wien · Heidelberger Platz 3, D-1000 Berlin 33
175 Fifth Avenue, New York, NY 10010, USA
37-3, Hongo 3-chome, Bunkyo-ku, Tokyo 113, Japan

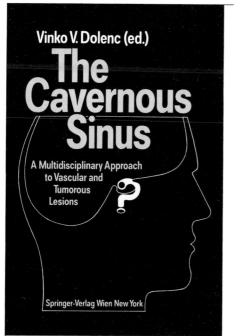

Vinko V. Dolenc (ed.)

The Cavernous Sinus

A Multidisciplinary Approach to Vascular and Tumorous Lesions

Springer-Verlag Wien New York

1987. 195 figures. IX, 419 pages.
Cloth DM 240,—, öS 1680,—.
ISBN 3-211-82000-0

Contents:
Historical Review and Pioneer Work
Anatomy
Diagnostic Procedures
Occlusions Techniques
Surgery of Vascular Lesions
Tumor Surgery.

The management of vascular and tumorous lesions of the parasellar region still remains one of the most demanding task in neurosurgery. It is only a short time ago that the major concepts of the anatomy of the so-called cavernous sinus were described in detail.

The book stresses that the improved understanding of normal structure and function of the cavernous sinus makes risk-free and effective operative treatment of intracavernous aneurysms, carotid-cavernous fistulas and tumors possible. It gives a view of our present understanding of the structure and function of the cavernous sinus and presents results and possibilities of the treatment of parasellar pathologies.

This stimulating book is the first comprehensive and up-to-date text dealing with the cavernous sinus and is addressed to anyone who is concerned with the diagnosis and treatment of lesions of the skull base.

Springer-Verlag Wien New York

Moelkerbastei 5, A-1010 Wien · Heidelberger Platz 3, D-1000 Berlin 33
175 Fifth Avenue, New York, NY 10010, USA
37-3, Hongo 3-chome, Bunkyo-ku, Tokyo 113, Japan